Ministry of Agriculture, Fisheries and Food

Manual of Nutrition

Eighth edition prepared by
David Buss and Jean Robertson

London: Her Majesty's Stationery Office

© Crown copyright 1976
First published 1945
Eighth edition 1976
Sixth impression 1982 (with amendments)

Contents

12 Nutritional value of meals

Tables

Foreword

This booklet is designed to give the reader a basic understanding of the science of nutrition. Some previous knowledge of a related field such as domestic science, food science, chemistry, biochemistry, or physiology would be useful but, as far as possible, this has not been assumed.

Nutrition may be learned (or taught) in a number of ways depending not only on previous knowledge but also on aptitudes and the time available. This Manual first describes the energy-producing nutrients and how they are obtained from our great variety of foods by digestion and absorption into the body, and then covers the minerals and vitamins. It continues with a discussion of all the main foods and many factors which affect their nutritional value, and ends with a guide for meal planning (including the cost) and the needs of special groups of people. There are also a number of useful Appendices, such as tables of the composition of selected foods, an outline of relevant UK legislation, and some suggestions for further reading. Previous editions of the Manual of Nutrition have often formed the basis for courses taught in this way.

Alternative approaches start from familiar foods, grouping them in a variety of ways according to their nutritional value. Once such example could be, a 'milk' group (including cheese and ice cream), a 'meat' group (including poultry, fish, eggs and perhaps cheese and legumes), a 'vegetable and fruit' group, and a 'bread and cereals' group. The number of servings of each to be taken each day and the nutritional reasons for this can be adapted to other cultures, and are comparatively easy to understand. Another way is to plan diets around a central core of carefully chosen cheap and nutritious foods. Alternatively foods may be grouped as 'energy-giving', 'body-building', and 'protective' according to the nutrients which predominate, as in the diagram:

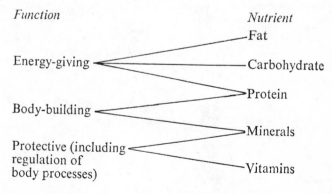

The information necessary for instruction organized in these ways can also be found in this Manual.

The booklet has been extensively revised in the Ministry's Nutrition Section in order to include a number of new items without increasing the total length; this should help to keep the price within everyone's reach. It is hoped that this edition will prove as useful as the previous ones developed from the material first organized by Dr Magnus Pyke in the Ministry of Food during World War II, and we would welcome suggestions for improvement.

Ministry of Agriculture, Fisheries and Food
April 1976

For this printing, a substantial number of small changes have been made to the nutrient content ascribed to certain foods. This is to make the values in this Manual as compatible as possible with those in the 4th edition of McCance and Widdowson's table of food composition. (See also Appendix 2.)

Ministry of Agriculture, Fisheries and Food
November 1977

PART 1

Nutrients and their utilization

1 Introduction to Nutrition, and some definitions

The foods eaten in other countries are very different from our own, yet the majority of people grow well and stay healthy provided that they get enough to eat. The reasons for this, and the ways in which the adequacy of any diet can be assessed, form part of the science of nutrition with which this Manual is concerned. A knowledge of its principles is thus important to all of us, but especially to those who plan and provide meals.

Before proceeding further, it is necessary to define some terms:

The science **Nutrition** is the study of all processes of growth, maintenance and repair of the living body which depend upon the digestion of food, and the study of that food.

Food is any solid or liquid which when swallowed can supply any of the following:

(a) material from which the body can produce movement, heat, or other forms of energy,
(b) material for growth, repair, or reproduction,
(c) substances necessary to regulate the production of energy or the processes of growth and repair.

Foods are considered in more detail in Part 2.

The components of foods which have these functions are called **nutrients.** They are introduced below, and considered in more detail in Chapters 2, 3, 4, 7 and 8.

The **diet** consists of those foods or mixtures of foods in the amounts which are actually eaten (usually each day). A **balanced diet** contains adequate amounts of all the nutrients.

The nutrients in food

The following types of nutrients may be present in foods:

Carbohydrates, which provide the body with energy, and may also be converted into body fat.

Fats, which provide energy in a more concentrated form than carbohydrates, and may also form body fat.

Proteins, which provide materials (amino acids) for growth and repair. They can also be converted into carbohydrate and used to provide energy.

1

Minerals, which are used in growth and repair, and help to regulate body processes.

Vitamins, which help to regulate body processes.[1]

Although water, like oxygen from the air, is also essential for life, it is not usually considered as a food or a nutrient. On the other hand, alcohol would be considered a food because it provides energy, even though it has drug-like properties. Iron from a cooking pot is also a nutrient since it may be used to renew substances in the blood.

Hardly any foods contain only one nutrient. Most are very complex mixtures, which consist mainly of a variety of carbohydrates, fats and proteins, together with water. Minerals and vitamins are present in very much smaller amounts. One hundred grams (g) of potatoes, for example, contain about 18 g carbohydrates, 2 g proteins, 80 g water, and less than 50 milligrams of the minerals and vitamins (and if fried they will also contain fat).

Energy

Energy is the ability to do work, and therefore means more than just vigorous activity. It can be derived from carbohydrates, fat, protein and alcohol not only in the body but also by burning them. Experiments show that almost exactly the same amount of energy is produced from, say, wheat when it is used for fuel in a railway engine (as it has been in times of glut) as when it is eaten by man. The essential difference between the two chemical processes is that in the body the energy is released gradually by a series of steps, each carefully controlled by an enzyme.[2] This energy is used to perform muscular work and to maintain body temperature and such processes as breathing, but a considerable amount is also lost as heat.

---

[1]*Vitamins* differ from hormones (which also help to regulate body processes) in that with the exception of vitamin D, they cannot be made in the body and must therefore be supplied in the diet; hormones are always made within the body itself.

[2]*Enzymes* are special proteins, each of which accelerates the rate of a specific chemical reaction without itself being affected. They enable complex changes to occur in the body that would otherwise require more extreme conditions; without them life could not exist. Many require the presence of vitamins or minerals as 'co-factors' in order to act.

Other constituents of food

Water

Water comprises about two-thirds of the body's weight, and is the medium or solvent in which almost every body process takes place both inside and outside the cells. The need of the body for water is second only to its need for air: man can survive for many weeks without food but for only a few days without water. Water comes from solid foods as well as from drinks (page 100), and it is lost by evaporation in the breath and sweat as well as in the urine. The balance of water retained in the body is normally very carefully regulated by the kidneys, but excessive losses can result from vomiting or diarrhoea in illness or from heavy sweating due to strenuous activity or a hot climate. Then, if water intake is not increased, dehydration may result. In temperate climates at least 1 litre (2 pints) of water or other fluid should be drunk each day; more will be needed if heavy work is done.

Fibre

Some foods, particularly whole cereals and some fruit and vegetables, contain substantial amounts of 'fibre' (roughage). In contrast to the nutrients described, this mixture of indigestible materials is not absorbed into the body; instead, it adds bulk to the faeces. This property may be beneficial to health, although fibre also decreases the absorption of certain nutrients – especially some of the minerals.

Flavours, colours, etc

In addition to the main nutritive and structural components, foods also contain innumerable minor constituents which give them their characteristic flavours and colours. Control over the changes which occur in these constituents after ripening, and during storage, preparation and cooking is an important part of the art of both cooks and food technologists.

Malnutrition

The maintenance of health in an individual depends upon the consumption and absorption of appropriate amounts of energy and all the nutrients. Too little or too much of some over a period of months may lead to malnutrition. Although the body has considerable power to adapt to reduced dietary intakes, for example by reduced physical activity, too low an intake of food will eventually result in *undernutrition,* and, in extreme cases, *starvation.* An example is the wasting (marasmus) in young children, and stunting of physical and perhaps even mental development, which may result from a poor weaning diet or from the poor diet of the mother. Excessive fatness, or *obesity,* resulting from too great a food intake, is also a form of malnutrition. Other examples include the 'classical' nutritional *deficiency diseases* such as scurvy and some anaemias which result from diets containing too little of one or more minerals or vitamins, or from a physiological inability to absorb these nutrients.

Standard measurements of amount

Standard units must be used to calculate the energy and nutrients in various amounts of food, and to measure heights and weights. Both the metric system (including the form known as SI[1]) and traditional units have been used in this edition of the Manual. The relationships between these units are given in some detail in Appendix 1.

---

[1]This system mainly affects the definition of energy, which has been measured in kilo*calories* (1 kcal being the amount of heat required to raise the temperature of 1 kilogram of water by 1°C). The SI unit, the *joule,* is hard to define in familiar terms, but 1 kilojoule (kJ) may be visualized as the amount of heat required to raise the temperature of 239 grams of water by 1°C.

2 Carbohydrates

There are three major groups of carbohydrates in food: *sugars, starches,* and *cellulose and related materials.* All are compounds of carbon, hydrogen and oxygen only, and their chemical structures are all based on a common unit (nearly always glucose). The units can be linked together in different ways and in different numbers, and classification of the carbohydrates depends primarily on the number of units; this varies from one to many thousands. Sugars and starches are a major source of man's food energy throughout the world.

Sugars

MONOSACCHARIDES (or simple sugars)

Glucose occurs naturally in fruit and plant juices and in the blood of living animals. Most carbohydrates in food are ultimately converted to glucose during digestion. Glucose can also be manufactured from starch by the action of acid or specific enzymes. *Glucose syrup* (liquid glucose) results from the partial hydrolysis of starch (usually maize or corn starch), and is a mixture of glucose, maltose and several more complex sugars. Although glucose is the sugar present in the highest concentration, this syrup is less sweet than pure glucose and is used in some manufactured foods such as sugar confectionery.

Fructose occurs naturally in some fruit and vegetables and especially in honey. It is the sweetest sugar known. It is also a component of sucrose, from which it may be derived, and is present in commercial 'high fructose' syrups.

Galactose does not occur in the free state, but forms part of lactose.

DISACCHARIDES

Disaccharides consist of two monosaccharides linked together (minus the elements of water):

5

Sucrose occurs naturally in sugar cane and sugar beet, and in lesser amounts in fruits and some roots such as carrots. It is a chemical combination of glucose and fructose. Refined sugar is essentially pure sucrose.

Maltose is formed during the breakdown of starch by digestion and, for example, when grain is germinated for the production of malt liquors such as beer. It is a combination of 2 glucose units.

Lactose occurs only in milk, including human milk. It is less sweet than sucrose, and is a combination of glucose and galactose.

Properties of sugars

All sugars, whether monosaccharides or disaccharides, dissolve in water and are varyingly sweet in taste. Their taste may be modified by cooking (e.g. by caramelization). They usually form white (colourless) crystals when the water in which they are dissolved becomes supersaturated, but impure preparations may be brown. In addition to providing a readily available source of energy and sweetness, sugars have other uses in foods: in jam-making, canning and freezing they act as preservatives, and in soft drinks and some other foods they help to provide a characteristic consistency.

Non-sugar sweeteners

Some other substances also taste sweet. *Sorbitol*, which is made from glucose and is related to the sugars, is sometimes used in diabetic foods because it is absorbed only slowly; however, its energy value is similar to that of glucose. In contrast, *saccharin* has no chemical or nutritional relationship to sugars and provides no energy. It does not rank as a food, but may be used as a sweetening agent when it is desirable to restrict the amount of sugar in the diet. It is about 500 times as sweet as sucrose.

Starch

There are a number of starches, which are POLYSACCHARIDES composed of variably large numbers of glucose units linked together to form both straight and branched chains (*amylose* and *amylopectin* respectively). They exist in granules of a size and shape characteristic for each plant. In this form they are insoluble in water so foods such as flour and potatoes are not usually eaten raw, but when heated or cooked in the presence of water the starch granules swell and eventually gelatinize. They can then be more easily digested.

Glycogen is similar to starch in composition, but is made from glucose only by animals and not by plants. Small amounts are stored in the liver and muscles as an energy reserve. It is not a significant item in the diet because it breaks down again to glucose after an animal's death.

Cellulose and related materials

These POLYSACCHARIDES provide the rigid and fibrous structure of vegetables, fruits and cereal grains (as well as wood), including the cell walls which enclose the starch granules. They are insoluble in water.

Cellulose consists of many thousands of glucose units. It cannot be digested by man, but can be used as food by cows and other ruminants whose digestive tract contains micro-organisms capable of breaking it down into glucose. Cellulose and certain other indigestible polysaccharides, collectively known as dietary fibre or roughage, add bulk to the faeces because of their water binding capacity and greatly assist the passage of digestible materials and waste products through the intestines. There is renewed interest in the relationship between this property and human health.

Pectin is another complex polysaccharide present in apples and many other fruits and in such roots as turnips. Its property of forming a stiff jelly is important in jam-making.

Sources of carbohydrates in the diet

Plants form sugars in their leaves by the action of sunlight, but store them in their stems, roots, tubers or seeds as starch (the small amount in unripe fruits, however, turns back into glucose on ripening). Starch forms the major energy reserve of most plants, and thus in turn provides a major part of man's food energy. Sugars would hardly be present in the diet at all except for lactose from milk and fructose from fruit and honey, were it not for the liberal use of sucrose, both alone and in jams, tinned fruit, cakes, biscuits, ice cream and other processed foods.

The sugar and starch content of selected foods is shown in Table 1. About one-third of the present intake of carbohydrate in the UK consists of sucrose, 7 per cent is lactose, and the remainder, starch; a century ago, flour and potato consumption was much higher and sucrose consumption much lower. Then, as in developing countries now, starch was even more important in the diet. The total fibre content of the average UK diet has not changed much over the past century, but a greater proportion now comes from fruit and vegetables and less from cereals as a result of changing eating habits.

Table 1. **Average carbohydrate content of some raw foods, g per 100 g (Available carbohydrate, as monosaccharides)**

	Sugars	Starch	Total
Milk	4.7[1]	0	4.7[1]
Ice cream	21.2	1.6	22.8
Meat	0	0	0
Sugar	105.3[2]	0	105.3[2]
Syrup	79.0	0	79.0
Jam	69.2	0	69.2
Potatoes	0.5	20.3	20.8
Beans, baked	5.2	5.1	10.3
Oranges	8.5	0	8.5
Bananas	16.2	3.0	19.2
Peaches, canned	22.9	0	22.9
Bread, white	1.8	47.9	49.7
Bread, wholemeal	2.1	39.7	41.8
Flour, white	1.7	78.4	80.1
Oatmeal	0	72.8	72.8
Biscuits, chocolate	43.4	24.0	67.4
Soup, tomato	2.6	3.3	5.9
Orange squash, undiluted	32.2	0	32.2

[1] Lactose
[2] Equivalent to 100 g of sucrose:
   1 g disaccharide is equivalent to 1.05 g monosaccharide.
   1 g starch is equivalent to 1.11 g monosaccharide.

Health aspects of carbohydrates

Although all sugars and starches absorbed by the body provide similar amounts of energy, they have different physiological effects. An excessive consumption of sugar (sucrose) and sweets is associated with increased tooth decay, especially when eaten between meals and in a form which sticks to the tooth surface, but there is more controversy about the relationship between different dietary carbohydrates and the development of obesity, diabetes, heart disease, and bowel diseases. For these reasons it is useful to know the amounts of both starch and sugar in different foods, and they are shown separately in Table 1.

People with diabetes are usually advised to regulate the carbohydrate content of their diet (page 31).

Some individuals, particularly of non-white races, have a limited ability to digest lactose. 'Lactose intolerance' is not usually found in infants who depend on milk, but it may develop in later life; it results in digestive disturbances when the equivalent of a glass or more of milk is drunk.

3 Fats

Fats include not only 'visible fats' such as butter and margarine, cooking fats and oils, and the fat on meat, but also the 'invisible fats' which occur in milk, nuts, lean meat, and other animal and vegetable foods. They are a more concentrated source of energy than carbohydrates, and are the form in which much of the energy reserve of animals and some seeds is stored.

Like carbohydrates, fats are compounds of carbon, hydrogen and oxygen only, but the proportion of oxygen is lower. Chemically, food fats consist mainly of mixtures of *triglycerides*. Each triglyceride is a combination of three *fatty acids* with a unit of glycerol (glycerine), and the differences between one fat or oil and another are largely the result of the different fatty acids in each.

Fatty acids

Dozens of different fatty acids are found in nature. They differ in the

Table 2. **Percentage composition of fatty acids in raw foods**

| | Fat g per 100 g | Fatty acids, per cent of fat by weight[1] | | |
		Saturated	Monounsaturated	Polyunsaturated
Milk, cows'	3.8	60	32	3
Milk, human	4.2	48	39	8
Cheese, Cheddar	33.5	60	32	· 3
Eggs	10.9	31	39	11
Beef, average	22.0	42	47	4
Lamb, average	30.2	48	38	5
Pork, average	29.0	40	44	8
Chicken	17.7	33	45	15
Liver, average	8.1	32	19	22
Herring	18.5	20	50	18
Butter	82.0	60	32	3
Margarine, hard	81.0	37	45	14
Margarine, soft	81.0	31	43	23
Corn (maize) oil	99.9	16	29	49
Olive oil	99.9	14	70	11

[1] The total percentage of fatty acids is less than 100 because of the glycerol and other fatty compounds which are present. To calculate the total fatty acid content of a food, multiply the percentages of the various types of fatty acid by the amount of fat. Thus the total polyunsaturated fatty acid content of 100 g of beef is $\frac{4}{100} \times 22.0 = 0.88$ g.

number of carbon atoms and 'double bonds' which they contain. *Saturated* fatty acids have no double bonds and this makes them stable, while *polyunsaturated* fatty acids have two or more double bonds which react gradually with air and make the fat rancid. Most fats contain both types, as well as *monounsaturated* fatty acids, but in widely varying proportions depending on the source (Table 2). Large amounts of polyunsaturated fatty acids affect the physical as well as the chemical properties of the fats, making them liquid at room temperature (i.e., oils). Unsaturated fatty acids can be changed into saturated fatty acids by controlled treatment with hydrogen (hydrogenation), as when liquid oils are hardened in the manufacture of margarine. The more important fatty acids in foods are:

SATURATED FATTY ACIDS

Palmitic acid and *stearic acid,* which are major constituents of hard fats such as lard, suet and cocoa butter.

Butyric acid, which, although present in only small amounts in milk fat and butter, makes an important contribution to their taste. Free butyric acid is released when these fats become rancid.

UNSATURATED FATTY ACIDS

Oleic acid (monounsaturated, with one double bond) occurs in substantial amounts in all fats, and especially in olive oil where it provides 70 per cent of the total fatty acid content.

Linoleic acid (with 2 double bonds), which occurs in large amounts in vegetable seed oils such as maize (corn) oil and soya bean oil, and in small amounts in some animal fats such as pork.

Linolenic acid (with 3 double bonds), which occurs in small amounts in vegetable oils, especially linseed oil.

Arachidonic acid (with 4 double bonds), which occurs in very small amounts in some animal fats. It can be formed in the body from linoleic acid. Fatty acids with even more double bonds occur in fish oils.

Linoleic, linolenic and arachidonic acids are called *'essential fatty acids'* because they are required in small quantities for normal health but cannot be made within the body. Once called vitamin F, enough of these fatty acids should be present in the diet to provide about 1–2 per cent of the energy intake.

11

Properties of fats

Fats are solid at low temperatures and become liquid when they are heated. Oils are simply fats which are liquid at room temperature, usually as a result of their higher content of unsaturated fatty acids. Oils and fats do not dissolve in water, but may be *emulsified* with water by vigorous mixing as when butter and margarine are made. Emulsions usually separate unless materials such as egg constituents are added.

Fat makes an important contribution to the texture and palatability of foods. Furthermore, because it is digested comparatively slowly, foods rich in fat have a high satiety value (page 27).

Food fats usually contain small amounts of other fat-soluble substances, including flavour components and some of the vitamins. Animal fats may contain retinol (vitamin A) and vitamin D, and varying amounts of cholesterol, while vegetable fats may contain carotenes (which can be converted into vitamin A in the body) and vitamin E, but no cholesterol:

Table 3. **Average cholesterol content of some raw foods, mg per 100 g**

Milk	14	Liver, average	330
Cheese, Cheddar	70	Butter	230
Eggs	450	Margarine	0–50[1]
Beef	65	Vegetable oil	0
Chicken, light meat	69		

[1] Value depends on proportion of animal fat included.

The amount of energy obtained from all common fats is about the same, despite the different functions of many of the component fatty acids.

Mineral oils such as liquid paraffin, are chemically different from food fats and oils despite their similarity in appearance. They cannot be utilized by the body, but function as laxatives and will reduce the absorption of some nutrients.

Sources of fat in the diet

Vegetable sources In plants, fats are formed from carbohydrate. Thus, when seeds such as sunflower and cottonseed ripen, their starch content decreases as their fat content rises. Oil seeds such as these, and groundnuts (peanuts), coconuts, rape, palm and soya beans contain about 20–40 per cent of oil; they are among the chief sources of fat for the manufacture of margarine. The fat content of flour and other cereal products apart from oatmeal is generally low, as is the fat content of most vegetables and fruits. The proportion of each fatty acid present is normally characteristic of the plant, although it can sometimes be altered by genetic breeding.

Animal sources Animals, including man, store excess energy almost entirely in deposits of fat, the amount of which is very variable. As in plants, this fat can be made from carbohydrate – but the dietary carbohydrate can be starch, sugar or even (in cows and sheep) cellulose. Animals also lay down fat from their dietary fat; in this case the fatty acid composition reflects that of the diet, except for ruminants whose digestive processes normally make the fatty acids more saturated.

Fish such as herring, mackerel, pilchards, salmon, sardines, tuna and eels, are sometimes called *fatty fish*; the proportion of fat in them varies with the season of the year. *White fish* such as cod, haddock and plaice contain little fat except in the liver; this liver is also a rich source of vitamins A and D.

The fat content of many foods, especially meat, varies widely. Average values, and the main sources of fat in the UK diet, are shown in Table 4. The amount of fat in the diet tends to be higher in more affluent families and countries, and the proportion of fat in the UK diet has steadily increased for many years.

The average proportion of polyunsaturated to saturated fatty acids in the whole diet is about 0.2:1, but would be increased if some of the beef, lamb and dairy products were replaced by poultry, fish or vegetable oils (including margarines rich in polyunsaturated fatty acids, but excluding coconut and olive oils).

Table 4. **Average fat content of some raw foods, g per 100 g**

Milk	3.8	Butter	82.0
Ice cream	7.4	Margarine	81.0
Cheese, Cheddar	33.5	Low-fat spread	40.7
Cheese, cottage	4.0	Cooking oil	99.9
Eggs	10.9	Lard and dripping	99.1
Beef, average	22.0	Potatoes	0
Bacon	40.5	Peanuts, roasted	49.0
Chicken	17.7	Bread, white	1.7
Fish, white, filleted	0.7	Bread, wholemeal	2.7
Herring	10−25	Flour, white	1.2
Salmon, canned	8.2	Oatmeal	8.7

Main sources of fat in the diet are butter, margarine and other fats and oils, meat, and milk.

13

4 Proteins

All proteins are compounds of carbon, hydrogen and oxygen, but, unlike carbohydrates and fats, they always contain nitrogen as well. Most proteins also contain sulphur and some contain phosphorus. They are essential constituents of all cells, where they regulate the processes of living or provide structure. Protein must be provided in the diet for the growth and repair of the body, but any excess can be converted into glucose and used to provide energy.

Proteins consist of chains of hundreds or even thousands of amino acid units. Only about 20 different amino acids are used, but the number of ways in which they can be arranged is almost infinite. It is the specific and unique sequence of these units which gives each protein its characteristic structural and enzymatic properties.

Amino acids

It is convenient to divide amino acids into two types: *essential* and *non-essential*. *Essential* amino acids cannot be made in the body, at least in amounts sufficient for health, and must therefore be present in the food. *Non-essential* amino acids are equally important as components of all proteins in the body; they differ only in that it is possible for them to be made from any excess of certain other amino acids in the diet.

The 8 amino acids essential for *adults* are:

Isoleucine	Phenylalanine
Leucine	Threonine
Lysine	Tryptophan
Methionine	Valine

and another amino acid, histidine, is also essential for the rapidly growing *infant*.

The remaining amino acids which are widespread in proteins are:

Alanine	Glycine
Arginine	Proline
Aspartic acid	Serine
Cysteine	Tyrosine
Glutamic acid	

14

Animal and vegetable proteins

The overall proportions of amino acids in any single vegetable food (cereals, nuts and seeds, potatoes, or legumes such as peas and beans) differ from those needed by man. For example, wheat is comparatively low in lysine, maize is low in tryptophan, and legumes are low in methionine (Table 5). These proteins are therefore said to have low *biological values,* because the *quality* of a protein depends on its ability to supply all the essential amino acids in the amounts needed. Mixtures of such foods, however, complement each other and result in greatly enhanced values.

Most animal proteins (from meat, fish, milk, cheese and eggs) have a high biological value. The reason for this is that man is part of the animal kingdom; the proteins of animals are therefore more like those of man and can be utilized by us with the minimum of waste. In effect, animals have pre-selected with varying degrees of efficiency the plant amino acids which we need and have burned up the remainder for energy (page 31). Nevertheless, the nutritional advantages of animal foods over vegetable foods in practice lie more in the presence of associated nutrients such as vitamin B_{12}, iron and vitamin D than in the protein.

Because there is no way in which excesses of amino acids can be stored in the body, they will be most efficiently used if a complete assortment is supplied to the body at about the same time. This can be achieved by eating a mixed diet at each meal – provided that the total energy content of the diet is also adequate. Mixtures of animal and vegetable protein foods such as fish and chips, bread and cheese, breakfast cereals with milk, and beans on toast, therefore have a sound physiological basis.

Texturized vegetable protein

Because animals convert plant protein into their own muscle slowly and inefficiently (only 5–10 per cent being retained), meat is expensive. Ways have therefore been developed to concentrate or isolate the proteins from

Table 5. **Proportion of some essential amino acids in selected proteins, g per 100 g protein**

	Lysine	Methionine	Tryptophan
Milk, cows'	8.0	2.8	1.4
Eggs	6.2	3.2	1.8
Beef	9.1	2.7	1.3
Beans, soya	7.0	1.4	1.4
Peanuts	4.1	1.3	1.3
Wheat[1]	2.8	1.7	1.2
Maize[1]	3.0	2.1	0.7

[1] Some amino acids can be increased by genetic breeding.

a number of plants, especially soya beans, and convert them *directly* into products which resemble meat. Such texturized vegetable proteins, if suitably fortified with the most important minerals and vitamins which meat provides, such as iron, thiamin, riboflavin and vitamin B_{12}, can be used instead of meat and are acceptable to vegetarians (vegetarian diets are discussed on page 90).

It is also possible to isolate protein from micro-organisms such as yeasts and fungi, or otherwise inedible leaves, but these are only used as animal feeds.

Protein as a source of energy

The amount and type of protein in the diet will not exactly balance the requirements for growth, repair and maintenance: there will always be excesses of some amino acids, and usually an excess of total protein. These will be converted into glucose in the liver or be directly oxidized to provide heat and energy. Furthermore, if the energy available from the diet is insufficient to meet demands, this oxidation of the amino acids tends to take preference over their more fundamental use for rebuilding proteins. This is why it is important to ensure that diets contain sufficient energy in the form of carbohydrate and fat before expensive proteins are added, for only then can these proteins be properly utilized for those purposes for which no other nutrient can be substituted.

Properties of proteins

Some proteins dissolve in water and some in salt water, but some do not dissolve. This is exploited in the preparation of wheat gluten, when other proteins as well as starch are washed from the flour.

The action of heat on proteins is complex. Proteins such as the albumen in egg white harden or coagulate irreversibly when heated, but are still readily digested. Individual amino acids are little affected by normal cooking procedures, although some lysine may react with carbohydrates in the food (e.g., in the baking of bread) and methionine may sometimes be reduced. In the preparation of gelatin, however, when connective tissue from meat is boiled for many hours, *all* the tryptophan is destroyed.

The brown discoloration which sometimes develops during prolonged storage of concentrated or dried milk or dehydrated vegetables is due to complex reactions between lysine and the sugars of these foods (the Maillard reaction).

Sources of protein in the diet

About one-third of the protein in the average UK diet comes from plant sources and two-thirds from animal sources. The amount of protein in nuts and dried peas and beans is very high – about the same as in meat, fish and cheese. The proportion is diluted when these legumes are soaked in water, but they remain an excellent source of good quality protein. Cereals are also rich in protein; indeed wheat, maize and rice are the main sources of protein for many people in the world. The amount of protein in most root vegetables is small, but potatoes provide useful quantities; green and leafy vegetables, however, contain insignificant amounts. The concentration of protein in selected foods is shown in Table 6.

Table 6. **Average protein content of some raw foods, g per 100 g**

Milk, cows'	3.3	Potatoes	2.1
Milk, dried skimmed	36.4	Peas, frozen	5.7
Cheese, Cheddar	26.0	Beans, baked	5.1
Eggs	12.3	Beans, butter, dry	19.2
Beef, average	17.1	Apples	0.3
Lamb, average	15.9	Peanuts, roasted	24.3
Pork, average	16.0	Bread, white	7.8
Chicken	17.6	Bread, wholemeal	8.8
Cod	17.4	Flour, white	9.8
		Cornflakes	8.6

5 Energy needs and food consumption

Uses of energy

Energy, i.e., the ability to do work, is obtained from food by controlled oxidation of the carbohydrates, fat, protein and alcohol in the diet. It is necessary for three purposes: (a) to maintain life, (b) for voluntary activities, and (c) for special purposes such as growth, pregnancy and lactation. If more is obtained than is used in these ways, the excess can be stored in the body as fat tissue.

MAINTENANCE OF LIFE

Energy is required for breathing, the heartbeat, the maintenance of body temperature, and other involuntary activities including brain function. The amount needed can be measured in people at complete rest or asleep. The rate of this *basal* or *resting metabolism* is higher in relation to body size in infants and actively growing young children than in adults. After adolescence, the needs are proportional to the amount of lean tissue in the body; thus women tend to have lower resting metabolic rates than men both because they are lighter and because muscle generally forms a lower proportion of their body weight (and fat a higher proportion). The rate is also lower in old people, or in starvation, because of the reduction which occurs in lean tissue.

After food is eaten, extra heat is produced and more energy is needed to cover this. The amount varies with the food. Climate does not significantly affect the resting metabolism, but the rate does vary widely between apparently similar individuals because the efficiency of the body processes varies. Some average values are:

	Weight kg	Resting energy requirement kcal(MJ)/day	kcal(MJ)/kg/day
Infant, 1 year old	10	500 (2.1)	50 (0.21)
Child, 8 years old	25	1,000 (4.2)	40 (0.17)
Adult woman	55	1,300 (5.4)	25 (0.1)
Adult man	65	1,600 (6.7)	25 (0.1)

A man therefore needs about 1 kilocalorie (nearly 5 kilojoules) each minute just to keep alive. During 8 hours sleep, the resting requirement of 400–500 kcal (1.7–2.1 megajoules) is all that would be used, but during the remainder of the day the additional requirements of physical activity must be taken into account.

ACTIVITY

Whenever people move, they use extra energy. The heavier they are the more it takes, and strenuous activities of course require more energy than light ones. There are also substantial variations between apparently similar individuals. It is easier to measure the total energy expended (*including the resting metabolic energy*) during any activity than it is to measure the supplement for that activity, and some examples of these totals are shown for an *average 25 year old man* weighing 65 kg (10 stone):

Everyday activities	Average energy expenditure kcal/min	kJ/min
Sitting	1.4	6
Standing	1.7	7
Washing, dressing	3.5	15
Walking slowly	3	13
Walking moderately quickly	5	21
Walking up and down stairs	9	38

Work and recreation

Light

Most domestic work		
Golf		
Lorry driving	2.5–4.9	10–20
Light industrial and assembly work		
Carpentry, bricklaying		

Moderate

Gardening		
Tennis, dancing		
Cycling up to 20 km per hr	5.0–7.4	21–30
Digging, shovelling		
Agricultural work, non-mechanized		

Strenuous

Coal mining, steel furnace work		
Squash, cross-country running	7.5 and over	Over 30
Football, swimming (crawl)		

Additional energy is needed during *growth* to provide for the extra body tissue. However, even in babies which are rapidly laying down fat, the amount is small in comparison with the needs for maintenance and movement.

During pregnancy and lactation, all the infant's needs for energy (as for other nutrients, see page 87) must be supplied by the mother. A total of about 80,000 kcal (335 MJ) of extra food energy is needed during a *pregnancy,* mostly during the final months. Some of this is used to build up a store about 4 kg of fat in the mother which may be gradually drawn upon during *lactation,* but an additional intake of 500 kcal (2.1 MJ) per day from the diet is also recommended at this time (page 54).

Total energy requirements

The dietary energy required by an individual who is neither gaining nor losing weight exactly equals the energy expended on maintenance and physical activity. In practice this balance is achieved over periods of a few days, with remarkable accuracy: an excessive intake of only 10 kcal each day would be equivalent to a weight gain of about 1 lb (0.5 kg) every year.

The energy expended during a day can be estimated from the average values given above, taking into account the times spent on different leisure and occupational activities. Thus, a male sedentary worker such as a civil servant might expend 2,700 kcal (11.3 MJ) in a typical day, as follows:

	kcal	MJ
8 hr asleep at 1.1 kcal per min	530	2.2
8 hr at work		
5 hr sitting, at 1.4 kcal per min	420	1.8
3 hr standing and walking, at 2.5 kcal per min	450	1.9
8 hr non-occupational activities		
2 hr washing and light domestic activities, at 3.25 kcal per min	390	1.6
2 hr travelling, sitting, standing and walking quickly, averaging 3.0 kcal per min	360	1.5
3 hr sitting, eating, watching television at 1.4 kcal per min	250	1.0
1 hr exercise or gardening at 5.0 kcal per min	300	1.3
Total energy expenditure	2,700	11.3

Because of individual variations, the diet of any particular sedentary worker may provide more or less energy than this; the average intake of a group of such people would, however, be expected to be close to this value.

In summary, the daily energy requirement of any adult is that amount which results in no long-term change in body weight. Energy requirements depend on:

Body size and composition Heavy people use more energy for maintenance and physical activity, although some may spend less time than lighter people in activities. Women tend to need less energy than men, although their needs are increased during pregnancy and lactation.

Age Requirements for maintenance are *proportionately* highest in infants and young children, and lowest in old people who have less lean body tissue and are less active.

Physical activity The degree of activity is the most important factor in determining energy requirements, and also the most difficult to assess. Sedentary workers (clerks, professional people, drivers and many shop assistants) need a total of about 900 kcal (3.8 MJ) for 8 hours work; moderately active workers (most industrial workers, railwaymen, postmen and bus conductors) need about 1,200 kcal (5.0 MJ) and very active workers (miners at the coal face, and some building labourers, farm workers, dockers, and army recruits) have an average need for about 1,800 kcal (7.5 MJ) during 8 hours at work. Leisure activities, particularly if indulged for long periods, also affect the day's requirements.

Obesity

If an individual eats or drinks foods which provide more energy than he uses up in his daily activity, some of the fat, protein, carbohydrate or alcohol will be converted into body fat. Any kind of food can therefore be 'fattening'. Some foods, however, are more concentrated sources of energy than others, or their palatability is such that excessive amounts are more likely to be eaten; these tend to be foods containing little water and a high proportion of fat or sucrose, such as butter, margarine and fried foods, and sugar, sweets, cakes and biscuits. Alcoholic drinks in excess can also lead to obesity, as appetite, which normally limits food intake, appears to restrict drinking somewhat less.

Life insurance companies have calculated desirable weights for people of different heights, their interest arising from the toll taken by obesity-related diseases including coronary heart disease, diabetes and complications arising during surgery:

Table 7. **Desirable weights for adults of medium frame**

| | Height (in bare feet) | | | Weight (without clothes) | |
	ft	in	cm	lb	kg
Men	5	5	165	122–135	55–61
	5	6	168	126–139	57–63
	5	7	170	130–144	59–65
	5	8	173	134–148	61–67
	5	9	175	138–152	63–69
	5	10	178	142–157	65–71
	5	11	180	146–162	66–74
	6	0	183	150–167	68–76
	6	1	185	154–172	70–78
	6	2	188	159–177	72–80
	6	3	191	164–182	75–83
Women	5	0	152	102–114	46–52
	5	1	155	105–117	48–53
	5	2	157	108–121	49–55
	5	3	160	111–125	50–57
	5	4	163	115–130	52–59
	5	5	165	119–134	54–61
	5	6	168	123–138	56–63
	5	7	170	127–142	58–65
	5	8	173	131–146	60–66
	5	9	175	135–150	61–68
	5	10	178	139–154	63–70

[Prepared from data published by the Metropolitan Life Insurance Company, 1959.]

The values in Table 7 are *not* increased during middle and old age.

Weight may be lost by decreasing energy intake, or increasing physical activity, or both. Conversely, weight may be gained by increasing energy intake or decreasing physical activity. The exact consequences of these changes are difficult to predict because of the large differences between individual responses, but the part played by changes in activity is likely to be comparatively small. For example, if a man trying to lose weight takes a brisk half hour walk, he will expend about 100 kcal (420 kJ) more than if he sat watching television. If at the end of his walk he is thirsty and drinks a pint of beer, he will take in substantially more energy than he used up and should not be surprised if his weight increases! Nevertheless, *regular* exercise can be an important factor in weight control.

Energy value of food

The energy provided by the fat, protein and carbohydrate in food, and by alcohol, can be measured. Taking into account the small proportions of these nutrients which are not absorbed into the body, it is accepted that:

1 g dietary carbohydrate (calculated as monosaccharides) provides 3.75 kcal or 16 kJ

1 g dietary fat provides 9 kcal or 37 kJ

1 g dietary protein provides 4 kcal or 17 kJ

1 g alcohol provides 7 kcal or 29 kJ

In some fruits and fruit products, small amounts of energy are derived from organic acids such as citric acid.✳Minerals, vitamins and, of course, water do not provide energy.

The energy value of any food can therefore be calculated when the proportions of these nutrients in it are known. For example, each 100 g white bread contains 7.8 g protein, 1.7 g fat and 49.7 g carbohydrate, so the energy content is calculated as follows:

$$7.8 \times 4 = 31.2 \text{ kcal from protein}$$
$$1.7 \times 9 = 15.3 \text{ kcal from fat}$$
$$49.7 \times 3.75 = 186.4 \text{ kcal from carbohydrate}$$
$$\text{Total} \quad 232.9 \text{ kcal}$$

or

$$7.8 \times 17 = 132.6 \text{ kJ from protein}$$
$$1.7 \times 37 = 62.9 \text{ kJ from fat}$$
$$49.7 \times 16 = 795.2 \text{ kJ from carbohydrate}$$
$$\text{Total} \quad 990.7 \text{ kJ}$$

It is misleading, however, to imply that energy values can be obtained with such precision; decimal points should not be included in the results, which might be rounded to 233 kcal or 990 kJ. But, when performing further calculations such as for the proportion of energy derived from protein, it is wiser to use the detailed figures and round off only at the end:

$$\frac{132.6}{990.7} \times 100 = 13.38 \text{ or } 13 \text{ per cent of the energy from protein.}$$

Sources of energy in the diet

Nearly all the weight of any food is made up of protein, fat and carbohydrate together with water. Foods which contain large amounts of water,

✳ NOTA BENE

such as salad vegetables, fruit and clear soups will contain little protein, fat or carbohydrate, and consequently provide little energy. In contrast, foods rich in fat (each gram of which provides more than twice as much energy as each gram of protein or carbohydrate) will be excellent sources of energy. The main sources of energy in the UK diet are bread, flour and other cereals, sugar, meat, visible fats and dairy produce – foods which are not only rich in energy but also eaten in substantial quantities. For some people, sweets and alcoholic drinks are also a significant source of energy. The energy (and water) contents of selected foods are shown in Table 8.

Table 8. **Average energy value and water content of some raw foods, per 100 g**

	Energy		Water
	kcal	kJ	g
Milk	65	272	87
Cheese, Cheddar	406	1,682	37
Eggs	147	612	75
Beef	266	1,107	64
Bacon	422	1,744	41
Chicken	230	954	65
Fish, white	76	322	82
Herring	234	970	64
Butter, margarine, average	735	3,020	16
Cooking oil	899	3,696	0
Sugar	394	1,680	0
Potatoes	86	369	76
Lettuce	9	36	96
Mushrooms	7	31	92
Oranges	35	150	86
Apples	46	196	84
Bananas	76	326	71
Dates	248	1,056	15
Bread, white	233	991	39
Flour, white	350	1,493	13
Biscuits, chocolate	524	2,197	2
Beer, bitter	31	129	94

The significance of hot foods

The heat of hot food is trifling compared with the energy provided by metabolism of its constituents within the body. For example, the constituents of tomato soup provide 55 kcal per 100 g; a serving of 250 ml (9 oz) would therefore provide about 140 kcal. The additional heat provided by its cooling from a serving temperature of, say, 60°C to the body temperature of 37°C would be about 6 kcal. Nevertheless, this heat is immediately perceived, and gives a useful boost to morale on cold days.

6 Digestion of food and absorption of major nutrients

Food has been defined as any solid or liquid which, when swallowed, can provide the body with energy, or material for growth and repair, or certain substances for regulating body processes. However, it is clear that almost any food can be recovered virtually intact from the stomach if vomiting occurs soon after it is eaten. Therefore, food cannot really be said to have entered the body until it has been:

(a) *Digested*, i.e., physically and chemically broken down into simple component parts which can be
(b) *Absorbed*, i.e., passed through the walls of the digestive tract into the blood (or lymph).

Flavour and appetite

For food to be eaten, it must be appetizing or we must be hungry or preferably both circumstances apply. When and how much we eat is determined by a number of factors. The complex sensation of *hunger* occurs when the body's energy stores are reduced (giving rise to reduced levels of glucose and fatty acids in the blood) and the stomach is empty.

But people, especially obese people, do not eat only when they are hungry and stop when they cease to feel hungry. *Appetite* is a sensation which relates to the smell and taste of particular foods, and is influenced by the surroundings, habits, and emotional state of the individual, all of which can also increase or decrease the flow of saliva and other digestive juices. Thus, where there is freedom of choice, more attractive food is more likely to be eaten, and it can be seen that good cooking and pleasant surroundings are important in nutrition. It should, however, be noted that some appetizing foods such as confectionery products can be relatively low in many nutrients, and that unappetizing foods can provide nourishment if they are eaten – as when an unconscious person is fed through a stomach tube.

The process of digestion

Although cooking softens meat fibres and the cellulose of plant materials, and gelatinizes starch, true digestion only begins when food enters the digestive tract. The digestive tract is illustrated in the diagram; it is basically a tube about 5 metres long.

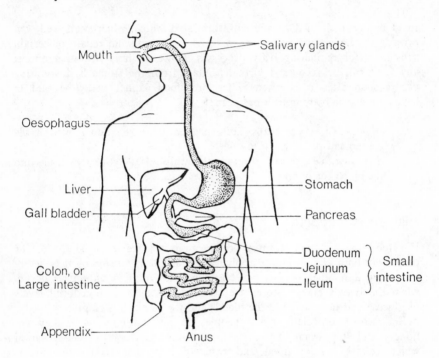

Diagram of Digestive System

In the mouth

(a) Food is mechanically broken down by chewing. It is therefore important to have healthy teeth and gums.

(b) The food is mixed and moistened with saliva.

Saliva comes from salivary glands under the tongue and at the back of the mouth. It is usually present in the mouth, but its flow is increased by the smell and taste of food and by chewing. It helps the food to be swallowed, and also contains an enzyme, ptyalin, which converts a small amount of the starch into maltose.

In the stomach

After the mixture of food particles and saliva has been swallowed – the final voluntary action – it takes about 3 seconds to pass down the oesophagus (gullet) into the stomach, where:

(a) The food is mixed with gastric juice.

(b) More mechanical breakdown results from stomach contractions.

Gastric juice is produced by the lining of the stomach in response to the same stimuli that increase saliva flow. Normally, about 3 litres are produced each day. It has three important constituents:

(a) The enzyme pepsin, which begins the digestion of protein.

(b) About 0.2 to 0.4 per cent of hydrochloric acid (much more acid than in 'acid foods') which destroys most of the bacteria which could be present in food and water and provides the acid conditions necessary for the pepsin to be active.

(c) 'Intrinsic factor', necessary for subsequent absorption of vitamin B_{12}.

Speed of digestion in the stomach The main purpose of the stomach is to act as a reservoir: digestion still proceeds if the stomach is completely removed. Food normally remains there for 2 to 4 hours before the resulting semi-liquid mixture (chyme) is passed by degrees into the small intestine. The exact time depends on the emotional state of the person and the type of food eaten: foods rich in carbohydrate (such as rice) pass most quickly and those rich in fat most slowly. The latter therefore delay the return of hunger longest, and are said to have a high satiety value.

In the small intestine

Despite its name, the small intestine is the longest part of the digestive tract. It is about 3 metres in length (although, because of the loss of tone and elasticity, it is found to be 7–8 metres long after death), compared with about 1 metre for the large intestine. It is, however, only 2–4 cm in diameter compared with 6 cm for the latter. The first distinct part of the small intestine is called the *duodenum*; the remainder consists of the *jejunum* and finally the *ileum*. It is in this organ that the main part of both digestion and absorption takes place.

In the duodenum, the digestive juices poured on to the food mixture from three sources are:

(a) *Bile,* which is produced in the liver and stored in the gall bladder. Bile salts emulsify the fat into microscopic droplets so that it can be digested.

(b) *Pancreatic juice,* from the pancreas. This alkaline liquid neutralizes the acid chyme, and contains a number of enzymes for breaking down fats, proteins and carbohydrates into much simpler substances. The most important of these are *lipase* which splits fatty acids from the triglycerides of fat, *trypsin* and *chymotrypsin* which split proteins into small peptides and amino acids, and *amylase* which splits starch into maltose.

(c) *Intestinal juice,* from the walls of the small intestine itself. This also contains digestive enzymes.

The final phase of digestion occurs *in* the intestinal wall after absorption, when peptides are split into their component amino acids, maltose is converted into glucose by *maltase,* sucrose into glucose and fructose by *sucrase,* and lactose into glucose and galactose by *lactase.*

In the large intestine

Substances which have resisted digestion thus far can be used for food by the bacteria present in the large intestine (colon). Some cellulose and other components of dietary fibre may then be broken down, and the bacteria will form B-vitamins and vitamin K which provide small amounts of additional nutrients for absorption.

Table 9. **Summary of the major enzymes of digestion**

	Where active	Action
Ptyalin (from saliva)	Mouth	Some starch to maltose
Pepsin	Stomach	Protein to peptides
Rennin (in infants only)	Stomach	Milk protein to peptides
Trypsin (from pancreas)	Intestine	Protein to peptides and amino acids
Chymotrypsin (from pancreas)	Intestine	Protein to peptides and amino acids
Lipase (from pancreas and intestine)	Intestine	Fat to fatty acids
Amylase (from pancreas)	Intestine	Starch (and glycogen) to maltose
Maltase	Intestinal wall	Maltose to glucose
Sucrase	Intestinal wall	Sucrose to glucose and fructose
Lactase	Intestinal wall	Lactose to glucose and galactose

Digestion in infants

Before birth, infants are nourished through their bloodstream via the mother's placenta. The change to intestinal digestion does not develop fully for several months. Three consequences in particular may be noted:

(a) For a few days, some whole proteins can be absorbed without digestion. In this way, antibodies against some diseases may be absorbed intact from the mother's milk.

(b) The stomach contains the enzyme *rennin,* which clots the casein of milk and begins its digestion.

(c) Starch cannot readily be digested until the infant is several months old.

Indigestion

A food or food component is indigestible if it cannot be fully broken down into substances capable of absorption. Some, such as lactose from milk in lactose-intolerant individuals, will reach the large intestine and be fermented by the bacteria present; this results in the production of gas and diarrhoea. Indigestion also means discomfort or pain in the gastro-intestinal tract resulting from eating. It can result as much from emotional factors as from the passage of indigestible foods.

The process of absorption

In the mouth

No significant absorption occurs through the lining of the mouth.

In the stomach

The following simple substances can pass through the lining of the stomach into the blood stream in *small* quantities:

(a) Water

(b) Alcohol

(c) Sugars

(d) Minerals which are soluble in water, such as salt

(e) Vitamins which are soluble in water, i.e., B-vitamins (but not vitamin B_{12}, which is absorbed in the ileum with the aid of the intrinsic factor produced by the stomach) and vitamin C.

In the small intestine

Almost all the absorption of nutrients occurs through the walls of the small intestine. Most of the water, alcohol, sugars, minerals, and water-soluble vita- are absorbed here, as well as the digestion products of the energy producing nutrients – that is:

(a) Peptides and amino acids from proteins

(b) Fatty acids from fats

(c) Disaccharides from starch

Fat-soluble vitamins are absorbed in association with the fatty acids.

Absorption into the cells of the intestinal wall is remarkably efficient; indeed, more than half of the small intestine can be removed without major consequences. The surface of the wall contains innumerable projections, called *villi*, which present a very large surface area (20–40 square metres in total) for absorption. This process occurs both passively (by diffusion) and actively (when specific nutrients are drawn into cells already containing large amounts of those nutrients).

Absorption can, however, be impaired. For example, substances such as laxatives or dietary fibre which speed the passage of the intestinal contents may reduce absorption in general, and the fibre and phytic acid present in wholemeal cereals may also reduce the absorption of specific minerals such as calcium, iron and zinc.

In the large intestine

The main purposes of the large intestine are to absorb water from the residue moving through it from the small intestine, and to store the resultant faeces until they are expelled through the anus. Faeces consist of the indigestible materials of food together with debris from the continuously replaced cells of the intestinal wall. The entire passage of food from mouth to anus takes from 1 to 3 days, but it can be decreased by disease or increased to as long as a week by diets very low in fibre.

The fate of major nutrients in the body

Carbohydrates

The disaccharides entering the intestinal wall are split into monosaccharides which are carried by the bloodstream directly to the liver. They may then be:

(a) Passed as glucose to all the cells of the body to be used directly for energy via a series of controlled steps which also produce carbon dioxide and water.

(b) Converted into glycogen and stored in the liver and skeletal muscles as a readily available source of energy.

(c) Converted into fatty acids and stored in the body fat (adipose tissue) as a source of energy.

Fats

Almost all the fatty acids which enter the intestinal wall are immediately
rebuilt into triglycerides which are carried to the bloodstream by lymph.
Fat, in the form of microscopic particles called *chylomicrons*, gives the
blood plasma a milky appearance for some time after a large meal is
eaten. Fat may be further transformed by the liver, and is finally deposited
in the adipose tissue. This reservoir of fat is constantly available as a
source of energy via another series of controlled steps which also gives rise
to carbon dioxide and water.

Proteins

When the peptides enter the intestinal wall they are split into amino
acids which are carried in the blood directly to the liver. Then:

(a) They may be passed into the general circulation where they enter
the body's 'pool' of essential and non-essential amino acids. These
are then built into the structural proteins and specific enzymes
which each cell needs.

(b) The excess of some amino acids may be converted into certain
others.

(c) The residual excess of amino acids is oxidized for energy, in some
cases after conversion into glucose. Urea is also formed and excreted
through the kidneys. If the diet as a whole is inadequate in energy,
then a greater proportion of the protein will be used for this purpose in order to keep the body alive.

Control of nutrients in the blood

Blood is the means by which most nutrients are carried to and from
the cells where they are needed. The concentration of most nutrients in
the blood is normally controlled automatically; thus when carbohydrate
is eaten, the resulting slight increase in blood glucose is soon reduced by
the hormone insulin. In *diabetes*, however, the pancreas does not secrete
sufficient insulin, and the blood glucose concentration increases until the
excess is excreted by the kidneys into the urine. In juvenile-onset diabetes,
the symptoms resulting from this imbalance are so severe that insulin
must be taken, but maturity-onset diabetes can usually be controlled by
dietary regulation leading to a reduction in body weight.

7 Minerals

Most if not all of the inorganic elements or minerals can be detected in the body, but only about 15 of them are known to be essential and must be derived from food. Minute amounts of a further 5 or more are necessary for normal life in other animal species, and may yet prove to be necessary for man; it is impossible, however, to conceive of a dietary deficiency of these.

Minerals have three main functions:

(a) As constituents of the bones and teeth. These include *calcium, phosphorus* and *magnesium*.

(b) As soluble salts which help to control the composition of body fluids and cells. These include *sodium* and *chlorine* in the fluids outside the cells (e.g., blood), and *potassium, magnesium* and *phosphorus* inside the cells.

(c) As essential adjuncts to many enzymes, and other proteins such as haemoglobin which are necessary for the release and utilization of energy. *Iron* and *phosphorus*, and most of the other elements described at the end of this chapter, act in this way.

The seven elements above are the best understood, and are in general needed in the greatest amounts in the diet or are present in the largest amounts in the body tissues (Table 10); these, together with sulphur which is mainly present as part of the amino acids methionine and cysteine, may be considered as the *major minerals*. The remainder, including cobalt, copper, chromium, fluorine, iodine, manganese and zinc, are equally essential but needed in smaller or much smaller quantities; they are called *trace elements*. A large excess of some of these such as copper can be poisonous.

MAJOR MINERALS

Iron

Function, and effects of deficiency

Healthy adults contain about 3 to 4 g of iron, more than half of which is in the form of haemoglobin, the red pigment of blood. Iron is also present

Table 10. Daily intake and total body content of minerals for a reference man

	Daily intake		Total body content	
Major minerals				
Calcium	1.1	g	1,000	g
Phosphorus	1.4	g	780	g
Sulphur	0.85	g	140	g
Potassium	3.3	g	140	g
Sodium	4.4	g	100	g
Chlorine	5.2	g	95	g
Magnesium	0.34	g	19	g
Iron	16.0	mg	4.2	g
Trace elements				
Fluorine	1.8	mg	2.6	g
Zinc	13.0	mg	2.3	g
Copper	3.5	mg	72	mg
Iodine	0.2	mg	13	mg
Manganese	3.7	mg	12	mg
Chromium	0.15	mg	Less than 2 mg	
Cobalt	0.3	mg	1.5 mg	

Intakes are generally likely to be far greater than requirements. A variable proportion is actually absorbed into the body (ranging from almost 100 per cent for sodium and chlorine down to about 5–10 per cent for iron, copper, manganese and probably chromium and cobalt too); the amount absorbed normally balances the amount lost in urine and sweat, except where increased retention is necessary during growth.

in the muscle protein myoglobin, and is stored to some extent in organs such as the liver. This store is an important source of iron for the first 6 months of an infant's life because the amount of iron in milk is small. Iron is involved with the use of oxygen: haemoglobin transports oxygen from the lungs to the tissues, and other iron-containing substances utilize the oxygen within the cells.

If food provides insufficient iron to replace the body's losses, the stores are gradually depleted. Eventually, anaemia results. Anaemia can also arise from a number of other causes including deficiencies of folic acid and vitamin B_{12}; cures are best effected medically and not nutritionally, for example by the use of iron salts which can be absorbed in much larger amounts than the iron from food.

Absorption and excretion

The amount of iron in the body is controlled almost entirely by the amount absorbed, because losses occur only when blood or other whole cells are lost in the general wear and tear of life. Losses do not occur at the end of the red blood corpuscles' life of 3–4 months, because the iron from them is efficiently re-utilized.

The absorption of iron from food is generally low, but is increased when the body's stores are depleted and when needs are greatest as in growing children or menstruating or pregnant women. Iron is most readily absorbed from meat including offal (up to 25 per cent). Only 5 per cent or less of other forms of iron such as those in eggs and vegetables or added to flour is absorbed; the exact amounts depend on other factors in the diet, e.g., it is increased by vitamin C.

Sources

About a quarter of the iron in the UK diet comes from meat. The total amounts of iron present in selected foods is shown in Table 11.

Table 11. **Total iron content of some raw foods, mg per 100 g**

Milk	0.1	Potatoes	0.5
Eggs	2.0	Cabbage	0.6
Beef	1.8	Watercress	1.6
Corned beef	2.9	Apricots, dried	4.1
Chicken	0.7	Bread, white	1.7
Liver, average	11.4	Bread, wholemeal	2.5
Kidney	6.0	Flour, white	2.4
Fish, white	0.3	Cornflakes	0.6
		Cocoa powder	10.5
		Chocolate, plain	2.4
		Wine, red	0.9

Main sources of iron in the diet are meat, bread, flour and other cereal products, potatoes and vegetables.

Calcium

Function, and effects of deficiency

Calcium is the most abundant mineral in the body. All but about 1 per cent of it is in the bones and teeth together with more than three-quarters of the body's phosphorus as calcium phosphates deposited in an organic framework. In addition to giving strength, these minerals act as a reserve supply for other needs and the calcium is constantly withdrawn into and replaced from the blood at carefully controlled rates. The remaining 5–10 g of calcium are essential for the contraction of muscles including the heart muscle, for nerve function, for the activity of several enzymes, and for normal clotting of the blood.

Too little calcium *in the bodies* of young children results in stunted growth and in rickets (where the leg bones are deformed); in women who lose large quantities of calcium through repeated pregnancies and lactation and in some old people the deficiency may show as osteomalacia (decalcified bones). Old people, especially women, also frequently develop osteoporosis (loss of bone). However, in Britain these diseases are unlikely to be caused by low levels of calcium *in the diet* for the body can normally adapt to these; the primary deficiency in rickets and osteomalacia is of vitamin D, so that too little calcium is absorbed (page 50), while the basic cause of osteoporosis is still unknown.

Absorption and excretion

Only 20–30 per cent of the calcium in the diet is normally absorbed and the remainder is lost in the faeces. But without adequate amounts of vitamin D, little or no calcium can be absorbed, and when fibre or phytic acid (present mainly in the outer layers of cereals) is added to the diet, calcium absorption is also reduced. It was partly to compensate for this that calcium carbonate was added to the high extraction flour used during and after World War II; it is still added to all flour except wholemeal even though it is now known that the body can adapt to the presence of phytic acid.

Excretion of the absorbed calcium is mainly through the kidneys, and it is increased when the diet contains large amounts of protein; some calcium is also lost in sweat. Adults normally absorb enough calcium to balance these losses until middle age unless they are immobilized, but pregnant and lactating women and growing children who are forming new bone must of course obtain more.

Sources

Few foods besides milk and cheese and, in Britain, most bread (page 75) contain significant amounts of calcium, as shown in Table 12. It is therefore important that these foods are included in the diet, especially for children and pregnant and lactating women whose needs are greatest.

Table 12. **Calcium content of some raw foods, mg per 100 g**

Milk, liquid	120	Potatoes	8
Milk, evaporated	280	Cabbage	57
Milk, dried skimmed	1,190	Watercress	220
Yogurt, natural	180	Apples	4
Cheese, Cheddar	800	Bread, white	100
Eggs	52	Bread, wholemeal	23
Beef	8	Flour, white	150
Fish, white	16	Rice	4
Sardines, canned	550		

Main sources of calcium in the diet are milk, cheese, bread and flour (if fortified) and green vegetables. For some people, hard water and the bones in canned sardines and salmon can be important sources.

Phosphorus

Phosphorus is the second most abundant mineral in the body and, in the form of various phosphates, has a wide variety of essential functions. Calcium phosphates provide the strength of the bones and teeth, and inorganic phosphates are a major constituent of all cells. Phosphates play an essential role in the liberation and utilization of energy from food. They are also constituents of nucleic acids and some fats, proteins and carbohydrates, and must be combined with some B-vitamins in the body before the latter can be active.

Because phosphorus is present in nearly all foods, dietary deficiency is unknown in man. Furthermore, phosphates are added to a number of processed foods. It should, however, be noted that high intakes of phosphorus in the first few days of life may produce low levels of calcium in the blood, and muscular spasms (tetany). This can result from the use of cows' milk which has a high ratio of phosphorus to calcium compared with human milk, and in which the calcium may combine with the fat present and be poorly absorbed.

Table 13. **Phosphorus and magnesium content of some raw foods, mg per 100 g**

	Phosphorus	Magnesium
Milk	95	12
Cheese, Cheddar	520	25
Eggs	220	12
Beef, average	150	17
Chicken	160	20
Cod	170	23
Potatoes	40	24
Cabbage	54	17
Oranges	24	13
Peanuts, roasted	370	180
Bread, white	97	26
Bread, wholemeal	230	93
Marmite	1,700	180

Magnesium

Most of the magnesium in the body is present in the bones, but it is also an essential constituent of all cells and is necessary for the functioning of some of the enzymes which are involved in energy utilization.

Magnesium is widespread in foods, especially those of vegetable origin because it is an essential constituent of chlorophyll. Less than half is normally absorbed and, unlike the chemically related element calcium, this process is unaffected by vitamin D. Deficiency is rare and, results from excessive losses in diarrhoea rather than from low intakes.

Sodium and Chlorine

Functions, and effects of deficiency and excess

All body fluids contain salt (sodium chloride), but especially those outside the cells such as blood. These elements are involved in maintaining the water balance of the body, and sodium is also essential for muscle and nerve activity.

Salt requirements are closely related to water requirements, and too low an intake results in muscular cramps. Salt intake may, however, have to be restricted in certain kidney diseases or where there is marked water retention. Very young infants also cannot tolerate high sodium intakes because their kidneys cannot excrete the excess, so salt should not be added to infants' diets. It is possible that habitually high salt intakes are associated with high blood pressure.

Absorption and excretion

It is essential for life that the concentration of sodium and chloride in the blood is maintained within close limits. As an excess of (added) salt in the diet is readily absorbed, control of sodium in the blood is achieved by its excretion through the kidneys into the urine. There is also a variable and uncontrolled loss through sweat. This is only significant after strenuous exercise or in hot climates, as for miners in deep pits, steel workers and athletes; extra salt will then be needed to prevent muscle cramps.

In a temperate climate the amount of salt needed by an adult is about 4 g per day, although this amount could be lost in the sweat in 3 hours of strenuous activity in the sun. Such an intake can be achieved from the salt already present in food, but most people add more and take in from 5 to 20 g per day.

Sources

Sodium and chlorine are comparatively low in all foods which have not been processed, but salt is added to very many manufactured foods. For example, salt is low in pork and other fresh meats but high in bacon, sausages and most meat products; low in herrings but high in kippers. Salt is also added to canned vegetables and most butter, cheese, bread and some breakfast cereals during manufacture, and to many foods during cooking and on the plate.

Potassium

Function, and effects of deficiency

Potassium is present largely in the fluids within the body cells where its concentration is carefully controlled. The total amount in the body can be measured, and is closely related to the amount of lean tissue. Potassium has a complementary action with sodium in the functioning of cells.

As with sodium, most of the potassium in the diet is absorbed and the excess is excreted through the kidneys. Losses may be large if diuretics or purgatives are frequently taken, and in diseases such as kwashiorkor where tissue breakdown as well as diarrhoea occurs. In severe cases of potassium depletion, heart failure may result unless supplements are given.

Table 14. **Sodium and potassium content of some raw foods, mg per 100 g**

	Sodium	Potassium
Milk	50	140
Cheese, Cheddar	610	120
Eggs	137	136
Beef, average	53	280
Pork, average	63	274
Bacon	1,480	233
Chicken	70	260
Liver, average	84	315
Kidney, average	197	263
Haddock, fresh	120	300
Herring	67	340
Kipper	990	520
Butter, salted	870	15
Margarine	800	5
Potatoes	7	568
Brussels sprouts	4	380
Cauliflower	8	350
Peas, fresh	1	342
Peas, canned, processed	330	170
Mushrooms	9	467
Oranges	3	197
Peaches, canned	1	151
Prunes, dry	12	864
Cornflakes	1,160	99
Coffee, instant	41	4,000
Marmite	4,500	2,600
Milk chocolate	120	420

The main sources of sodium in the UK diet are table salt, bread and cereal products, meat products including bacon and ham, and milk. The main sources of potassium are vegetables, meat and milk. Fruit and fruit juices are also noteworthy as being much richer in potassium than sodium.

TRACE ELEMENTS

Knowledge of the exact roles and dietary requirements for several of the following minerals is incomplete for three reasons: they have only recently been found to be essential; dietary deficiencies of many are unknown; and the utilization of one may be affected by the amounts of other elements present.

Cobalt

Cobalt can be utilized by man only in the form of vitamin B_{12} (page 47).

Copper

Copper is associated with a number of enzymes. Deficiency has occasionally been observed in malnourished infants, particularly if their initial stores were depleted by prolonged feeding of cows' milk alone (which contains less copper than most foods).

Chromium

Chromium is involved in the utilization of glucose.

Fluorine

Fluorine is associated with the structure of bones and teeth, and increases the resistance of the latter to decay. Drinking water is an important source, but the natural content is variable and is often below the optimum level of 1 mg per litre (1 part per million). The only other important sources of fluorine in the diet are tea and sea-food, especially fish whose bones are eaten.

Iodine

Iodine is an essential constituent of hormones produced by the thyroid gland in the neck. Deficiency causes this gland to enlarge – a condition known as goitre. The most reliable source of iodine is sea-food; the amount in animal foods depends on the level in the animals' diets, and the amount in vegetable and cereal foods depends on the level in the soil. The use of iodized table salt is beneficial in areas where goitre is prevalent, whether it results from low intakes of iodine or from reduced absorption caused by goitrogens in some green vegetables.

Manganese

Manganese is associated with a number of enzymes. Tea is exceptionally rich in manganese, and plant products including nuts, spices and whole cereals are in general much better sources of manganese than are animal products.

Zinc

Zinc is also associated with the activity of a number of enzymes, but most of the comparatively large amount which is present in the body is in the bones. Zinc is present in a wide variety of foods, particularly in association with protein. Less than half of the zinc in the diet is absorbed, and absorption is further reduced if large amounts of whole cereals rich in fibre and phytic acid are eaten; this is as likely a cause of deficiency (resulting in stunting) as is a low intake *per se*.

8 Vitamins

Until the beginning of the 20th Century, it was believed that the only components of a diet necessary for health, growth and reproduction were pure proteins, fats, carbohydrates and a number of inorganic elements. This view had to be changed when it was found that minute amounts of additional materials were also essential. These factors could be extracted from a variety of foods, and appeared to be of two types: fat-soluble ('A') and water-soluble ('B'). They were later each discovered to contain several active components, or vitamins. The former, mainly associated with fatty foods, is now known to include vitamins A, D, E and K. The vitamin B complex includes thiamin (B_1), riboflavin (B_2), nicotinic acid (or niacin), folic acid, vitamin B_6, vitamin B_{12}, biotin and pantothenic acid. Vitamin C is also water-soluble, but occurs in different foods from the B-vitamins. Many of these vitamins exist in more than one chemical form.

The absence of a vitamin from the diet, or, more commonly in practice, its presence in insufficient amounts, leads to both general and specific symptoms. The most common general symptoms are, as with deficiencies of many other things, a feeling of malaise and restriction of the growth of children. The specific symptoms of deficiency in man are discussed separately for each vitamin. Excessive intakes of water-soluble vitamins, either from vitamin pills or from very unusual diets, have very little effect and are mostly excreted in the urine, but excessive intakes of fat-soluble vitamins accumulate in the body and can be dangerous.

Factors affecting the stability of the vitamins in foods are discussed elsewhere (page 62).

Vitamin A

The chemical name of vitamin A is *retinol*. Retinol itself is found only in animal foods, but milk and some vegetable foods also contain the deep yellow or orange *carotenes* which can be converted in the body to retinol and are therefore sources of vitamin A activity. The most important of these is beta(β)-carotene. The most convenient way of expressing the total vitamin A activity of a diet is as *retinol equivalents:* by definition, 1 μg retinol equivalent is equal to 1 μg retinol or 6 μg β-carotene[1] (except for milk where, because of better absorption, 2 μg β-carotene = 1 μg retinol equivalent). This takes into account the conversion losses and lesser absorption of β-carotene compared with retinol in the general diet.

Function, and effects of deficiency or excess

Vitamin A is essential for vision in dim light; thus prolonged deficiency (sufficient to deplete any stores in the liver, which in previously well nourished people will last for 1 to 2 years) results in night blindness. In children in many parts of the world deficiency also results in severe eye lesions (xerophthalmia) and complete blindness (keratomalacia). Vitamin A is also necessary for the maintenance of healthy skin and surface tissues, especially those which excrete mucus.

Excessive doses, for example from taking large amounts of vitamin A preparations for long periods, accumulate in the liver and can be poisonous.

Sources

Vitamin A is not widely distributed in food. Fish liver oils are by far the most concentrated natural source of retinol, but animal liver, kidney, dairy produce and eggs also contain substantial amounts; lard and dripping, however, contain none. Variable amounts of β-carotene are found in carrots and dark green or yellow vegetables, roughly in proportion to the depth of their colour; thus dark plants such as spinach contain more than cabbage, and the dark outer leaves of a cabbage contain more than the pale inner heart. Furthermore, all margarine for retail sale is required by law to contain about the same amount of vitamin A as butter. This is now added in the form of synthetic retinol and β-carotene.

The amounts of vitamin A in selected foods are shown in Table 15. The British diet as a whole provides on average about twice the recommended intake of vitamin A, with two-thirds coming from retinol itself and the remaining third from carotene.

---

[1]The amounts of vitamin A in foods are sometimes quoted in international units (i.u.). To convert these to μg retinol equivalents, multiply the i.u. of retinol (in animal foods) by 0.3, and divide the i.u. of β-carotene (in plant foods) by 10. (This is because 1 i.u. vitamin A = 0.3 μg retinol or 0.6 μg β-carotene; and 1 μg retinol equivalent = 1 μg retinol or 6 μg β-carotene.)

Table 15. **Vitamin A content of some raw foods, μg per 100 g**

Animal foods	Retinol
Milk	40[1]
Cheese, Cheddar	410[1]
Eggs	140
Beef	0
Liver, ox	16,760[1]
Kidney, average	120
Cod	0
Herring	45
Sardines, canned	0
Butter	985[1]
Margarine	900[1]
Cod liver oil	18,000
Halibut liver oil	900,000

Vegetable foods	β -Carotene	Retinol equivalent
Potatoes	0	0
Cabbage	300	50
Spinach	6,000	1,000
Peas, fresh or frozen	300	50
Watercress	3,000	500
Carrots, old	12,000	2,000
Tomatoes	600	100
Apricots, dried	3,600	600
Flour	0	0

[1] Retinol equivalent (including carotene).

Main sources of vitamin A in the diet are butter, margarine, liver, milk, green vegetables and carrots.

B-Vitamins

Although the chemical structure of each of the B-vitamins is quite different, they have several features in common. They act as 'co-factors' in different enzyme systems in the body; they tend to occur in the same foods; and, being water-soluble, they are not stored for long in the body. These characteristics mean that diets containing too little of the B-vitamins can lead to *multiple* deficiency diseases within a few months.

Thiamin (Vitamin B₁)

Function, and effects of deficiency

Thiamin is necessary for the steady and continuous release of energy from carbohydrate. Thiamin requirements are thus related to the amount of carbohydrate, and more or less to the amount of energy, in the diet. The deficiency disease, beriberi, results from a diet which is not only poor in thiamin but also rich in carbohydrate (or alcohol), such as one based almost entirely on polished rice from which the thiamin-rich seedcoat has been removed.

Sources

Thiamin is widely distributed in both animal and vegetable foods. Rich sources are those which contain more than 0.04 mg per 100 kcal (0.01 mg per 100 kJ), such as milk, offal, pork, eggs, vegetables and fruit, whole grain cereals and fortified breakfast cereals. It should, however, be noted that cooking may result in considerable losses from these foods (page 62). Fats and sugars contain no thiamin at all.

Wheat in the form of bread has long been a major source of carbohydrate in the British diet, but much of the thiamin is removed with the bran in the milling necessary to produce the popular white bread. Thus 1 oz of wholemeal bread provides 0.07 mg thiamin (0.10 mg per 100 kcal), while 1 oz of unfortified white bread would provide about 0.03 mg thiamin (0.04 mg per 100 kcal). It is therefore a legal requirement in the UK that all flour except wholemeal be *fortified* with thiamin to at least 0.24 mg per 100 g, equivalent to 0.07 mg per 100 kcal (page 75).

Table 16. **Thiamin content of some raw foods**

	mg per 100 g	mg per 100 kcal
Milk	0.04	0.06
Beef, average	0.05	0.02
Corned beef	0	0
Pork	0.59	0.18
Bacon	0.36	0.09
Sausages, pork	0.04	0.01
Sugar	0	0
Potatoes	0.11	0.13
Peas, fresh	0.32	0.48
Oranges	0.10	0.29
Peanuts, roasted	0.23	0.04
Bread, white	0.18	0.08
Bread, wholemeal	0.26	0.12
Oatmeal	0.50	0.13
Cornflakes, fortified	1.80	0.49
Marmite	3.10	1.80
Beer, bitter	0	0

Main sources of thiamin in the diet are bread and flour, meat, potatoes and milk.

Riboflavin (Vitamin B₂)

Function, and effects of deficiency

Riboflavin is a bright yellow substance, which is essential for the utilization of energy from food. Specific deficiency signs are rarely seen in man, but include sores in the corners of the mouth.

Sources

Although riboflavin is widely distributed in foods, especially animal foods, about one-third of the average intake in Britain is derived from one source alone – milk. As riboflavin will be destroyed by ultra-violet light, it is very important that milk is not allowed to stay too long on the doorstep.

Table 17. **Riboflavin content of some raw foods, mg per 100 g**

Milk	0.19
Cheese, Cheddar	0.50
Eggs	0.47
Beef, average	0.17
Chicken	0.14
Liver, average	3.10
Kidney, average	1.90
Potatoes	0.04
Bread, white	0.03
Cornflakes, fortified	1.60
Tea, dry	0.90
Marmite	11.0

Main sources of riboflavin in the diet are milk, meat (particularly liver) and eggs.

Nicotinic acid

Function, and effects of deficiency

Nicotinic acid and nicotinamide are two forms of another B-vitamin (known as niacin in the United States) which is involved in the utilization of food energy. Deficiency results in pellagra, in which the skin becomes dark and scaly especially where it is exposed to light.

Sources

Two anomalies occur with pellagra: it occurs when the diet consists largely of maize, a cereal which contains nicotinic acid, and it can be cured by milk or eggs which are not rich sources of this vitamin. The reasons are firstly, that the nicotinic acid in maize and other cereals is largely present in a bound form which is unavailable to man (although it can be released by alkali as in the preparation of Mexican tortillas), and secondly, that proteins of milk and eggs are especially rich in tryptophan – an amino acid which can be converted to nicotinic acid in the body.

It is therefore convenient to express the nicotinic acid content of foods in terms of equivalents: on average *1 mg of nicotinic acid equivalent equals 1 mg of available nicotinic acid or 60 mg of tryptophan,* and this is accepted as a definition. The amounts of both forms in selected foods is shown in Table 18.

Table 18. **Nicotinic acid equivalents in some raw foods, mg per 100 g**

	Nicotinic acid (total)	Tryptophan	Nicotinic acid equivalent[1]
Milk	0.1	47	0.9
Cheese, Cheddar	0.1	367	6.2
Eggs	0.1	217	3.7
Beef	3.7	218	7.3
Pork	4.1	178	7.0
Chicken	6.0	197	9.3
Fish, white	1.7	195	4.9
Potatoes	1.2	31	1.7
Peas, frozen	2.1	55	3.0
Bread, white	1.4	98	2.2
Bread, wholemeal	3.9	106	1.7
Tea, dry	6.0	0	6.0
Coffee, instant	22.0	186	25.1

[1] Available nicotinic acid + (tryptophan ÷ 60).
[2] Naturally occurring nicotinic acid is considered unavailable.

Main sources of nicotinic acid in the diet are meat and meat products, bread and flour, fortified breakfast cereals, vegetables and milk.

Vitamin B6 (Pyridoxine)

Function, and effects of deficiency

Vitamin B_6, or pyridoxine, is involved in the metabolism of amino acids, including the conversion of tryptophan to nicotinic acid; the requirements are thus related to the protein content of the diet. The vitamin is also necessary for the formation of haemoglobin. Pyridoxine deficiency once occurred in infants fed inadequate milk formulae, and women who are pregnant or taking oral contraceptives may benefit from increased intakes of this vitamin.

Sources

Vitamin B_6 occurs widely in food, especially in meats and fish, eggs, whole cereals and some vegetables.

46

Vitamin B_{12}

Function, and effects of deficiency

Vitamin B_{12} is a mixture of several related compounds, all of which contain the trace element cobalt. With folic acid, it is needed by rapidly dividing cells such as those in the bone marrow which form blood. Deficiency leads to a characteristic (pernicious) anaemia and to the degeneration of nerve cells. Because vitamin B_{12} does not occur in vegetable foods, deficiency may occur in vegans who consume no meat, milk, eggs, or any special supplement, but it more usually arises in those few individuals whose gastric juice contains none of the 'intrinsic factor' necessary for its absorption (page 29).

Sources

Vitamin B_{12} occurs only in animal products. Liver is the richest source, but useful amounts also occur in eggs, cheese, milk, meat and fish as shown in Table 19.

Table 19. **Vitamin B_{12} content of some raw foods, μg per 100 g**

Milk	0.3
Cheese, Cheddar	1.5
Eggs	1.7
Beef, lamb and pork	1.6
Liver, ox	110.0
Liver, lamb	84.0
Liver, pig	25.0
Fish, white	2.0
Marmite	0.5

Folic acid

Function, and effects of deficiency

Folic acid has several functions, including its action with vitamin B_{12} in rapidly dividing cells. Deficiency leads to a characteristic (megaloblastic) form of anaemia which must be distinguished from that caused by a deficiency of vitamin B_{12}. Folic acid deficiency can arise not only from a poor diet, as with some elderly people, but also because of increased needs for the synthesis of red blood cells in pregnant women and premature infants, and when there is decreased absorption of folic acid in gastrointestinal disease or when some anti-epileptic drugs are given.

Folic acid occurs in many foods, but is especially rich in offal and raw green leafy vegetables. Pulses, bread, oranges and bananas also provide folic acid, but other fruits, meat and dairy produce contain little. Folic acid is readily destroyed in cooking, much being lost in the water used for cooking vegetables; this, and the fact that some complex forms of folic acid are only partially broken down into free folic acid in the intestinal wall for absorption, means that care should be taken to include good sources of this vitamin in the diet.

Pantothenic acid

Pantothenic acid is necessary for the release of energy from fat and carbohydrate. Dietary deficiencies of this vitamin are unlikely in man because it is so widespread in food. Animal products, cereals and legumes are especially rich sources.

Biotin

Biotin is also essential for the metabolism of fat. Very small amounts are required, and sufficient may well be made by the bacteria normally inhabiting the large intestine. It is therefore probable that no additional biotin need be provided in the diet, except in the very unusual situation when large quantities of raw eggs are consumed: raw, but not cooked, egg white contains a substance (avidin) which combines with biotin making it unavailable to the body.

Rich sources of biotin include offal and egg yolk. Smaller amounts are obtained from milk and dairy products, cereals, fish, fruit and vegetables.

Vitamin C (Ascorbic acid)

Function, and effects of deficiency

Vitamin C is necessary for the maintenance of healthy connective tissue. Man is one of the few animals (along with monkeys and the guinea pig) unable to form his own vitamin C, and must therefore obtain it from food. Deficiency soon results in bleeding, especially from small blood vessels and into the gums, and wounds heal more slowly. Scurvy follows, and, if the deficiency is prolonged, death results. Mild deficiencies may occur in infants who are given unsupplemented cows' milk preparations, in people eating poor diets (particularly the elderly), and in food faddists eating little but whole cereals which contain no vitamin C.

Claims that extremely large amounts of vitamin C (10–100 times the recommended intake) prevent or cure colds and other minor ailments have little scientific basis.

Sources

Vitamin C is not widely distributed in foods. Small amounts occur in milk, especially breast milk, and liver, but virtually all the vitamin C in most diets is derived from fruit and vegetables. As many of these are difficult to store and are comparatively expensive when out of season, and since vitamin C is readily lost from them during storage, preparation and cooking (page 63), this vitamin remains one of the few nutrients in which British diets can be deficient.

The average vitamin C content of selected foods is shown in Table 20.

Table 20. **Vitamin C content of some raw foods, mg per 100 g (edible weight)**

Brussels sprouts	87
Cauliflower	64
Cabbage	53
Potatoes	
New	30
October, November	20
December	15
January, February	10
March to May	8
Tomatoes	20
Lettuce	15
Blackcurrants	200
Strawberries	60
Oranges	50
Lemon juice	50
Grapefruit	40
Apples	5
Pears	3
Plums	3

Main sources of vitamin C in the diet are potatoes, green vegetables and citrus fruit.

Some less commonly eaten fruits such as rose hips are even richer than blackcurrants or citrus fruits, but for practical reasons their extracts are now usually fortified with the equally valuable synthetic vitamin C. Vitamin C may also be added to other fruit juices to compensate for the losses which would otherwise occur during storage.

The amount of vitamin C in any particular fruit or vegetable may differ considerably from the value shown in the table. This is because of the natural variations which occur, and because of the losses during the time between harvesting and consumption in the home. As an example, fresh peas may contain between 10 and 30 mg per 100g; the higher values would tend to occur in the spring and early summer when the plants are growing most rapidly. The loss which can occur after harvesting

49

is illustrated in Table 20 by the average change in composition of potatoes through the year; it can also be substantial in the few days which elapse between the harvest of leafy vegetables and their consumption in the home. Vitamin C, like riboflavin, is also rapidly lost when milk is allowed to stand on the doorstep; this may be important for young children and those old people with restricted diets for whom milk may be one of the few sources of this vitamin.

The highest single contribution to vitamin C intake in the UK is made by potatoes (page 60), for the large amounts eaten more than compensate for the comparatively low content of this vitamin. The only vegetable materials containing no vitamin C are cereal grains (unless they are allowed to sprout) and dried peas and beans; instant potato also contains very little unless it has been fortified.

Vitamin D

Function, and effects of deficiency and excess

Vitamin D is necessary for maintaining the level of calcium (and phosphorus) in the blood. It achieves this primarily by enhancing the absorption of dietary calcium from the intestine, and by helping to regulate the interchange of calcium between the blood and bone.

Infants and children who obtain too little vitamin D develop rickets, with deformed bones which are too weak to support their weight. Because these changes readily become permanent, it is important to prevent their development; hence in the UK and some other countries vitamin D preparations are provided for children and pregnant women, and margarine and milk products are fortified. Some adolescents and women who are repeatedly pregnant and who breast-feed all their babies, and some old people, may also suffer from bone softening (osteomalacia) because they absorb too little calcium from a diet which is low in both calcium and vitamin D.

Too high an intake of vitamin D causes more calcium to be absorbed than can be excreted; the excess is then deposited in, and damages, the kidneys. It is therefore necessary for vitamin D intakes to be carefully controlled, especially in young children.

Sources

Vitamin D is obtained both from the action of sunlight on a substance in the skin, and from the diet. Sunlight is by far the most important source for most people, who will need little or no extra from food. But two groups of people should ensure that their food contains sufficient vitamin D: firstly, children and pregnant and lactating women, whose requirements are especially high, and secondly, people who are little exposed to sunlight such as the housebound elderly and people in northern latitudes or those who prefer to wear enveloping clothes.

Few foods contain vitamin D. All those which do so naturally are animal products, and contain vitamin D_3 (cholecalciferol) derived as in humans from the action of sunlight on the animal's skin or from its own food. There may thus be seasonal variations in the amounts present. Vitamin D_2 (ergocalciferol), which appears to be equally effective in man, can readily be manufactured from plant materials; it is added to some foods and is required by law in margarine for retail sale (page 67). Vitamin D is also included in the supplements provided (free to those in need) in the UK for pregnant and lactating women and for children up to 5 years old.

Table 21. **Vitamin D content of some raw foods, μg per 100 g**

Milk, liquid, winter	0.01
Milk, liquid, summer	0.03
Milk, UHT	0.02
Evaporated milk[1]	2.91
Cheese, Cheddar	0.26
Eggs	1.75
Liver, average	0.75
Herring and kipper	22.40
Salmon, canned	12.50
Sardines, canned	7.50
Butter	0.76
Margarine[1]	7.94
Ovaltine, dry[1]	30.60
Cod liver oil	212.50

[1] Includes added vitamin D.

Main sources of vitamin D in the diet are on average, margarine, fatty fish, eggs and butter. Each of these is, however, often unfortunately avoided by some people.

Vitamin E

Function, and effects of deficiency

A number of related *tocopherols* show vitamin E activity, the most active being alpha(α) – tocopherol. In rats it is necessary for normal fertility, but neither this nor many other wondrous properties ascribed to it have been proved in man. Because vitamin E occurs widely in foods, especially in those eaten by the poorest of the world's peoples, and because (like other fat-soluble vitamins) it is stored in the body, deficiency is only .likely in premature infants who have very low fat stores; when fed on formulas low in vitamin E and rich in the readily oxidized polyunsaturated fatty acids

51

which appear to increase the need for this vitamin, an anaemia may develop. Excessive intakes do not appear to be toxic.

Sources

Most foods contain vitamin E. The richest sources are vegetable oils, cereal products and eggs; animal fats and meat, fruit and vegetables contain comparatively little.

Vitamin K

Vitamin K is necessary for the normal clotting of blood. A dietary deficiency is unlikely, partly because the vitamin is widespread in vegetable foods such as spinach, cabbage and cauliflower, peas and cereals, and partly because our intestinal bacteria can synthesize it.

9 Recommended intakes of nutrients

An adequate intake of all nutrients is essential for health and activity, and there are additional requirements for growth, pregnancy, lactation and in times of stress such as infection. The exact amounts needed are different for each individual, and depend not only on such readily quantifiable factors as height, weight and sex, but also on physical activity throughout the day, the rate of internal activities such as heart beat, and the climate.

As these *requirements* can only be determined after lengthy experimentation, it is impracticable if not impossible to discuss what they are. Instead, a number of national and international bodies have *recommended* certain nutrient intakes for various groups of the population in question. These recommendations are designed to ensure that the needs of almost all healthy persons will be covered.

It follows that recommended intakes will always be higher than estimates of average requirements (except for energy, which is discussed below). Conversely, the actual nutrient requirements of almost all individuals will be less than the recommended intakes. Therefore, if a person's diet consistently contains more of a nutrient than is recommended he is almost certainly obtaining more than his requirement, but if it consistently contains less he may still be obtaining enough. But the further his intake falls below the recommendations, the greater his likelihood of malnourishment with its accompanying clinical symptoms.

Energy is different from other nutrients in that appetite normally controls the intake and keeps it close to requirements, and in that intakes in excess of requirements are undesirable and may lead to obesity. The recommendation for each *group* of people is therefore set at its estimated average requirement; about half of the *individuals* in the group will thus require more and half of them will require less than this.

Table 22 summarizes the daily intakes of energy and nine other nutrients which were recommended by the Department of Health and Social Security in a report published in 1979. They are believed to be sensible and practicable for the United Kingdom, but, like all such recommendations, will need to be revised in the light of new knowledge. Other essential nutrients were not discussed in the Report, but it is probable that requirements for these nutrients will be more than met if a good mixed diet is eaten in amounts which satisfy the needs for the major nutrients. Never-

Table 22. Recommended daily amounts of nutrients for population groups (DHSS, 1979)

Age ranges	Energy		Protein	Calcium	Iron	Vitamin A (retinol equivalent)	Thiamin	Riboflavin	Nicotinic acid equivalent	Vitamin C	Vitamin D[1]
years	MJ	kcal	g	mg	mg	μg	mg	mg	mg	mg	μg
Boys											
Under 1	3.25	780	19	600	6	450	0.3	0.4	5	20	7.5
1	5.0	1,200	30	600	7	300	0.5	0.6	7	20	10
2	5.75	1,400	35	600	7	300	0.6	0.7	8	20	10
3 – 4	6.5	1,560	39	600	8	300	0.6	0.8	9	20	10
5 – 6	7.25	1,740	43	600	10	300	0.7	0.9	10	20	—
7 – 8	8.25	1,980	49	600	10	400	0.8	1.0	11	20	—
9 – 11	9.5	2,280	56	700	12	575	0.9	1.2	14	25	—
12 – 14	11.0	2,640	66	700	12	725	1.1	1.4	16	25	—
15 – 17	12.0	2,880	72	600	12	750	1.2	1.7	19	30	—
Girls											
Under 1	3.0	720	18	600	6	450	0.3	0.4	5	20	7.5
1	4.5	1,100	27	600	7	300	0.4	0.6	7	20	10
2	5.5	1,300	32	600	7	300	0.5	0.7	8	20	10
3 – 4	6.25	1,500	37	600	8	300	0.6	0.8	9	20	10
5 – 6	7.0	1,680	42	600	10	300	0.7	0.9	10	20	—
7 – 8	8.0	1,900	48	600	10	400	0.8	1.0	11	20	—
9 – 11	8.5	2,050	51	700	12[2]	575	0.8	1.2	14	25	—
12 – 14	9.0	2,150	53	700	12[2]	725	0.9	1.4	16	25	—
15 – 17	9.0	2,150	53	600	12[2]	750	0.9	1.7	19	30	—
Men											
18 – 34 Sedentary	10.5	2,510	62	500	10	750	1.0	1.6	18	30	—
18 – 34 Moderately active	12.0	2,900	72	500	10	750	1.2	1.6	18	30	—
18 – 34 Very active	14.0	3,350	84	500	10	750	1.3	1.6	18	30	—
35 – 64 Sedentary	10.0	2,400	60	500	10	750	1.0	1.6	18	30	—
35 – 64 Moderately active	11.5	2,750	69	500	10	750	1.1	1.6	18	30	—
35 – 64 Very active	14.0	3,350	84	500	10	750	1.3	1.6	18	30	—
65 – 74	10.0	2,400	60	500	10	750	1.0	1.6	18	30	—
75 and over	9.0	2,150	54	500	10	750	0.9	1.6	18	30	—
Women											
18 – 54 Most occupations	9.0	2,150	54	500	12[2]	750	0.9	1.3	15	30	—
18 – 54 Very active	10.5	2,500	62	500	12[2]	750	1.0	1.3	15	30	—
55 – 74	8.0	1,900	47	500	10	750	0.8	1.3	15	30	—
75 and over	7.0	1,680	42	500	10	750	0.7	1.3	15	30	—
Pregnant	10.0	2,400	60	1,200	13	750	1.0	1.6	18	60	10
Lactating	11.5	2,750	69	1,200	15	1,200	1.1	1.8	21	60	10

[1] Most people who go out in the sun need no dietary source of vitamin D (p. 50), but children and adolescents in winter, and housebound adults, are recommended to take 10μg vitamin D daily.

[2] These iron recommendations may not cover heavy menstrual losses.

theless, the National Research Council of the United States has also recommended specific allowances for folic acid, vitamin B_6, vitamin B_{12}, vitamin E, magnesium, zinc, phosphorus and iodine in the 1974 edition of their 'Recommended Dietary Allowances', and the World Health Organization of the United Nations have considered a large number of additional trace elements. Some further points to be borne in mind are:

Energy The recommendations were based on the energy intake or expenditure of groups of the UK population, and refer to average or reference weights. Although there is normally no need for adjustment for groups of different weights, there is evidence that average energy intakes are now declining, perhaps in relation to our reduced energy expenditure.

The average value for infants under one year conceals the rapid growth which occurs during this time. The daily intakes recommended during the first year are:

	MJ	kcal	kcal/kg
Birth to 3 months	2.3	550	120
3 up to 6 months	3.2	760	115
6 up to 9 months	3.8	910	110
9 up to 12 months	4.2	1,000	105

Protein The intakes recommended are somewhat arbitrary, and represent 10 per cent of the energy requirement (e.g., for infants under one year, the 20 g protein recommended provides, at 4 kcal per gram, 80 kcal; this is 10 per cent of the recommended energy intake of 800 kcal). This level ensures a palatable diet and adequate provision of other nutrients which tend to accompany protein in foods, but man can consume much smaller quantities of protein and still retain good health. The latter amounts, including allowances for protein quality and the variation in physiological requirements, are given as the minimum requirements. It should, however, be noted that if energy requirements are not fully met at the same time, that protein which is eaten will be utilized more to provide the needed energy than for growth and tissue repair.

Fat and Carbohydrate There appears to be no absolute dietary requirement for either fat or carbohydrate, except for a small amount (1–2 per cent of energy requirements) of essential fatty acids. However, fat increases the palatability of the diet and in the UK it is unlikely to provide less than 30 per cent of the energy. The present intake of more than 40 per cent of energy requirements is considered by many authorities to be excessive. Some carbohydrate (50–100 g/day) is also necessary to prevent the undesirable effects which result from extremely high fat diets, and roughage is also important. Sucrose intakes should not be too high.

Calcium and Iron Both recommendations allow for the limited absorption of these nutrients from the diet.

Nicotinic acid and Vitamin A The intakes recommended allow for the likely contributions made by tryptophan and carotenes to the pre-formed nicotinic acid and retinol intakes respectively.

Vitamin C There are differing opinions as to the quantity of vitamin C required for health. It is generally agreed that 10 mg daily will not only prevent but also cure scurvy. The recommended intake of 30 mg is thought to provide a reasonable safety margin; there is no nutritional advantage from enormously higher intakes although there may be some pharmacological action.

Vitamin D It is not possible to make firm estimates of dietary needs because most of our requirements are met by vitamin D formed from the action of sunlight on a substance present in the skin. The amounts recommended may be considered as a safety measure for those who are little exposed to sunlight.

Excessive intakes of vitamin A and vitamin D accumulate in the body and are poisonous. Storage capacity for the other nutrients apart from energy (as fat) is limited; nevertheless the healthy body contains enough reserves to last for several weeks even if there were none in the diet. Thus, while recommended intakes are most conveniently expressed in daily terms, it is not necessary for the diet to contain these quantities *every* day. It is sufficient if the requirements are met over a period of, say, a week.

PART 2

Nutritional value of food and diets

The *nutritional importance* of a food in the diet depends upon:
(a) The composition of the raw food or ingredients as purchased
(b) The amount that is usually eaten
(c) The extent to which nutrients are lost during preparation or cooking.

Many factors combine to produce small variations in the nutrient content of a particular food crop or animal; *representative* values for the nutrient content of a wide selection of foods will be found in the tables in Appendix 2 (page 99) which should constantly be referred to when using this part of the Manual. Most people have individual preferences for certain foods and can use the tables to calculate the nutritional importance of these in their own diet.

Table 23, which is derived from the National Food Survey, provides a useful guide to the relative contributions of different foods to the average household diet in Britain, after allowance has been made for the expected losses of thiamin and vitamin C during cooking.

Cooking and processing

Most foods have to be prepared and cooked before they can be eaten. For some foods the process may be simple, as in the peeling of an orange. For others it may be complicated: for example wheat grains must be separated from the inedible parts of the plant and milled into flour, which in turn may need to be treated before being baked into bread. At each stage some of the nutrients will be discarded or destroyed, whether the process takes place in a factory or in the home. The nutrients may be further reduced if the food is stored for long periods, particularly if conditions are not ideal.

Although these losses are usually not of major significance if a good mixed diet is eaten (as this will still provide a considerable excess of nutrients over the recommended intakes) it is nevertheless desirable that the losses are kept to a minimum. A discussion of the main methods of cooking and preserving foods is therefore followed by descriptions of the factors which tend to reduce the stability of each nutrient. Applications to specific foods are discussed in Chapter 11.

Table 23. Percentage contribution made by groups of foods to the nutrient content of the average household diet

	Energy	Protein	Fat	Carbo-hydrate	Calcium	Iron	Vitamin A (retinol equivalent)	Thia-min	Ribo-flavin	Nicotinic acid equivalent	Vitamin C	Vitamin D
Milk (including cream)	13	20	15	7	51	4	14	14	36	12	9	12
Cheese	2	5	4	–	11	1	5	1	4	3	–	2
Total Milk, Cream and Cheese	*15*	*25*	*19*	*7*	*62*	*5*	*19*	*15*	*40*	*15*	*9*	*14*
Meat, carcase	6	11	12	–	} 2	11	1	7	6	14	–	–
Bacon and ham	3	3	6	–		1	–	4	1	2	–	–
Other meat and meat products	7	14	11	2	2	16	24	7	12	17	1	1
Total Meat	*16*	*28*	*29*	*2*	*2*	*28*	*25*	*18*	*19*	*33*	*1*	*1*
Fish	1	4	1	–	1	2	–	1	1	4	–	19
Eggs	2	5	3	–	2	5	3	1	8	4	–	16
Margarine	4	–	9	–	–	–	9	–	–	–	–	34
Butter	7	–	16	–	–	–	17	–	–	–	–	9
Other fats and oils	4	–	10	–	–	–	–	–	–	–	–	–
Total Fats	*15*	*–*	*35*	*–*	*–*	*–*	*26*	*–*	*–*	*–*	*–*	*43*
Sugar and Preserves	10	–	–	22	–	1	–	–	–	–	2	–
Potatoes	4	4	–	9	1	8	–	10	3	9	24	–
Green vegetables	} 4	2	–	1	2	4	4	3	2	2	17	–
Root vegetables		–	–	–	1	1	14	1	1	1	3	–
Other vegetables		3	1	3	2	7	5	3	2	3	8	–
Total Vegetables	*8*	*9*	*1*	*13*	*6*	*20*	*23*	*17*	*8*	*15*	*52*	*–*
Fresh fruit	1	} 1	–	2	1	1	} 1	2	1	} 1	20	–
Other fruit including nuts	1		1	3	1	2		1	1		14	–
Total Fruit	*2*	*1*	*1*	*5*	*2*	*3*	*1*	*3*	*2*	*1*	*34*	*–*
Bread and flour	17	19	2	31	16	22	–	26	3	13	–	–
Cakes, pastries, biscuits and other cereals	12	7	7	17	6	10	1	17	12	8	–	6
Total Cereals	*29*	*26*	*9*	*48*	*22*	*32*	*1*	*43*	*15*	*21*	*–*	*6*
Beverages and other food	2	2	2	3	3	4	2	2	7	7	2	1
Total	**100**	**100**	**100**	**100**	**100**	**100**	**100**	**100**	**100**	**100**	**100**	**100**

Home cooking

Heat is generally applied to food in one of three ways:

(a) Directly, with or without additional fat – as in roasting, grilling and baking (250–475°F; 120–250°C).
(b) With water – as in boiling, stewing and braising (212°F; 100°C).
(c) With fat – frying (310–435°F; 155–225°C).

Microwaves and infra-red cooking are mainly used for reheating and cooking frozen and fresh foods outside the home in snack bars, cafeterias and canteens. They cause relatively little additional destruction of nutrients.

Heat causes chemical and physical changes in food which in general make the flavour, palatability and digestibility of the raw product more acceptable and may improve its keeping quality. Heat may also increase the availability of some nutrients by destroying enzymes and anti-digestive factors. But cooking more usually results in the loss of nutrients, this being greatest at high temperatures, with long cooking times, or if an excessive amount of liquid is used. The losses of soluble vitamins and minerals are, of course, reduced if meat drippings and cooking water are not discarded but used in (for example) gravies.

Home freezing

This increasingly popular method of food preservation may result in some loss of thiamin and vitamin C when vegetables are blanched in water before freezing, but less than would otherwise result from the continuing action of enzymes in the plant tissues during storage. If the temperature of the freezer is kept below –18°C (0°F) there is almost no further loss of nutritional value until the food is thawed. In general, differences between the nutrient content of cooked fresh foods and cooked frozen foods as served on the plate are small.

Industrial processing

Processing in a factory is mainly intended to preserve food so that the choice is greater and independent of geographical area or the season of the year; it also reduces the time spent on preparing food in the home. The main commercial processes which cause some loss of nutrients are blanching, heat processing, and drying or dehydration. The *freezing* process itself has little effect on nutritional value, and since the delay after harvesting is minimal the nutrients in fresh foods are generally well retained.

Blanching or scalding in water or steam to minimize enzyme activity is a first step in the preservation of vegetables, whether by heat processing, freezing or dehydration. The process is carefully controlled, but small amounts of some minerals and water soluble vitamins dissolve in the water or steam and are lost.

Heat processing in metal cans or bottling in glass jars, will reduce the amounts of heat-sensitive vitamins, especially thiamin, folic acid and vitamin C. The losses will depend on the length of time needed to destroy any harmful organisms, and this will be greater for larger cans and in foods of a close consistency, such as ham, because of the slow transfer of heat from the outside to the centre. They will also depend on the acidity of the food and the presence of light and air; it is therefore difficult to give precise values for expected losses.

Dehydration (in air) in carefully controlled conditions has little effect on most nutrients, but about half the vitamin C is lost and there is a complete loss of thiamin if sulphur dioxide is added. Prolonged sun drying as in the production of raisins allows substantial changes to occur. Suitable packaging of dried foods is essential to prevent nutrient losses during storage.

Stability of individual nutrients

Protein is denatured by heat, and when cooking conditions are severe it will become less available for utilization within the body. This is partly because the changes in structure make the protein less readily digested and partly because some of the component amino acids will be destroyed – most notably lysine, which can react with carbohydrates in the food. These losses can also occur during prolonged storage even at room temperature.

Vitamin A Both retinol and β-carotene are stable to most cooking procedures, although at high temperatures and in the presence of air (e.g., when butter or margarine are used in frying) there will be some loss. Some loss also occurs in prolonged storage if light and air are not rigorously excluded.

The *B-vitamins* are all water soluble and most are also sensitive to heat.

Thiamin is one of the least stable of vitamins. It is readily dissolved out of foods into the cooking water and will be lost in the drippings from meat. It is fairly stable to heat if the food is acid, but the losses can be considerable under alkaline conditions, for example when sodium bicarbonate is added during cooking. It has been calculated that on average about 20 per cent of the thiamin content of all the food brought into the home is lost during cooking and reheating, but the loss is greater

62

in some foods than in others. Any foods which have been preserved by the use of sulphur dioxide, such as sausages and some potato products, will contain very little thiamin.

Riboflavin · will be lost in discarded cooking water and meat drippings; it is also unstable to alkali, and especially sensitive to light.

Nicotinic acid is an exceptionally stable vitamin, and will be lost only through its solubility in water.

Other B-vitamins All are soluble in water. Vitamin B_6, folic acid and panthothenic acid are also sensitive to heat, and can therefore be lost in cooking and canning.

Vitamin C is perhaps the least stable of all the vitamins. In addition to being water-soluble, it is very readily destroyed by air. This destruction is accelerated by heat, by alkali, and by the presence of certain metals, e.g., copper or iron. Vitamin C is also rapidly oxidized when an enzyme present in fruit and vegetables is released by any physical damage to the plant such as cutting. Thus poor cooking practices such as prolonged boiling of green vegetables in large amounts of water containing sodium bicarbonate to improve the colour, followed by keeping hot, can result in destruction of all the vitamin C originally present. Vitamin C is, however, partly protected by sulphur dioxide.

Vitamin D is stable to normal cooking procedures.

Vitamin E is not soluble in water and is stable to heat. It is, however, oxidized in the presence of air.

Table 24 summarizes the sensitivity of the most important nutrients.

Table 24. **Summary of factors ($\sqrt{}$) which may reduce the nutrients in food**

Nutrient	Heat	Light	Air	Water (by leaching)	Acid	Alkali	Other
Protein	$\sqrt{}$ if prolonged						
Minerals				$\sqrt{}$			
Vitamin A	$\sqrt{}$ with air		$\sqrt{}$ with heat				Metals
Thiamin[1]	$\sqrt{}$		$\sqrt{}$	$\sqrt{}$		$\sqrt{}$	Sulphur dioxide
Riboflavin		$\sqrt{}$		$\sqrt{}$		$\sqrt{}$	
Folic acid	$\sqrt{}$		$\sqrt{}$ (but protected by vitamin C)	$\sqrt{}$		$\sqrt{}$	
Vitamin C[1]	$\sqrt{}$		$\sqrt{}$ (but protected by sulphur dioxide)	$\sqrt{}$		$\sqrt{}$	Enzymes; metals

[1] Least stable to cooking and storage.

63

11 Foods

Milk

Importance in the diet

Cows' milk is the most complete of all foods, containing nearly all the constituents of nutritional importance to man; it is however comparatively deficient in iron and vitamins C and D. Unlike other foods of animal origin, milk contains a significant amount of carbohydrate, in the form of the disaccharide lactose (page 6).

Typical amounts of the major nutrients present *in one pint of liquid (pasteurized) milk* are given below; milk from the Jersey and Guernsey breeds of cows contains rather more fat.

	nutrients per pint
Energy	380 kcal
	1,592 kJ
Protein	19.3 g
Fat	22.2 g
Carbohydrate	27.5 g
Calcium	702 mg
Iron	0.6 mg
Vitamin A (retinol equivalent)	230 μg
Thiamin	0.23 mg
Riboflavin	1.11 mg
Nicotinic acid equivalent	5.3 mg
Vitamin C	9[1] mg
Vitamin D	0.13 μg

[1] As delivered to the home. This falls to 6 mg after 12 hours.

Average milk consumption is now about two-thirds of a pint per head daily; the contribution which this makes to the nutrient content of the average household diet is shown on page 60. It can be seen that in a mixed diet milk is particularly valuable for its content of high quality protein and easily assimilated calcium, and as a rich source of riboflavin; moreover, milk provides good nutritional value for money (page 86).

It is important that bottled milk is not left on the doorstep exposed directly to sunlight for a period of an hour or more, since a substantial amount of the riboflavin (and vitamin C) will be destroyed.

Effects of cooking

When milk is heated in the home the protein partially coagulates and forms with the fat a 'skin' on the milk surface; this holds the steam and causes the characteristic 'boiling over'. Food such as fish or vegetables, when baked in the milk, can also cause coagulation of milk proteins. Some caramelization of the sugars in milk may occur with long cooking in a very slow oven, as for example in milk puddings.

Effects of processing

When milk is *homogenized* the fat globules are broken up mechanically and distributed throughout the milk so that they no longer rise to the surface forming a creamy layer at the top of the milk bottle; the nutritional value of homogenized milk is similar to that of pasteurized milk.

Skimmed milk is milk from which most of the fat has been removed together with the fat-soluble vitamins A and D, but the amounts of protein, calcium and riboflavin are unchanged. It is most widely bought in the form of *instant dried skimmed milk powder*.

A variety of heat treatments are used to improve the keeping quality of liquid milk. The fat, fat-soluble vitamins, carbohydrates and minerals of milk are not affected by heat – but where the heat treatment is relatively harsh, slight changes occur in the availability of some of the amino acids in the milk proteins. The vitamins in milk which are partially destroyed by heat processing are vitamin C, thiamin, pyridoxine, vitamin B_{12} and folic acid.

Most of the liquid milk supply in Great Britain is *pasteurized*. During this mild form of heat treatment the milk is heated to about 72°C (162°F) for 15 seconds, killing any disease-causing bacteria. About 10 per cent of the thiamin and vitamin B_{12}, and 25 per cent of the vitamin C are destroyed, but in a mixed diet milk is not an important source of these nutrients. Very similar losses occur when milk is *spray dried*. The ultrahigh temperature (*UHT*) treatment of milk, in which a temperature of about 130°C (266°F) is maintained for one or two seconds, also causes some vitamin losses which are very similar to the losses in pasteurization. UHT milk packed aseptically into special containers which protect it from light and from oxygen will keep satisfactorily for several months without refrigeration, but variable losses of vitamin C and folic acid may occur during storage.

Sterilized milk is subjected to a more drastic form of heat treatment; it is prepared from homogenized milk which is bottled and then heated to about 120°C (248°F) for 20–60 minutes. About 60 per cent of the vitamin

C in the raw milk and 20 per cent of the thiamin are destroyed during the process.

Evaporated milk is prepared by the concentration of liquid milk at low temperatures; the milk is subsequently sterilized in cans at 115°C (239°F) for 15 minutes. In general, the nutrient losses are similar to those in sterilized milk.

Sweetened condensed milk is prepared similarly, but since it contains added sucrose the processing temperature needed for an adequate storage life is lower. Nutrient losses are therefore lower too, and are generally similar to those that occur in pasteurization.

Milk products

Cream

Cream is derived from fresh milk either by skimming off the fatty layer which rises to the surface or by spinning in a mechanical separator. Minimum fat contents for different types of cream are specified in Government Regulations; these include: single cream, 18 per cent by weight as milk fat; double cream, 48 per cent; whipping cream, 35 per cent; and clotted cream, 55 per cent fat. These compare with an average of 3.8 per cent fat in milk. The energy value of different types of cream varies directly with the fat content.

Yogurt

The nutritional value of yogurt is similar to that of the milk and minor ingredients used in its preparation, except that in products with added sugar the energy content is increased. The commercial product is based either on whole milk or on skimmed milk which is inoculated with a selected culture of lactic bacteria under controlled conditions. Dried skimmed milk may be added to produce a firmer consistency; flavourings, fruit juices, fruit and sugar are often incorporated to give a varied product. Some varieties of yogurt are fortified with vitamins A and D.

Butter

Butter is made by churning cream in a rotating drum so that the fat globules separate from the liquid buttermilk. In this country butter must contain not less than 78–80 per cent milk fat and not more than 16 per cent water. 1–2 per cent of salt is added to salted butter during manufacture. The amounts of vitamins A and D in butter are variable; representative values are shown in Appendix 2. **Margarine** is not a dairy product but a butter substitute made by homogenizing a mixture of oils and fats with brine. Almost any edible oils can be used for margarine and for low-fat spreads, as their physical properties can be modified first to give different proportions of polyunsaturated fatty acids (page 11). Vitamins A and D must by law be added to margarine for retail sale. The values required are 760 to 940 international units of vitamin A and 80 to 100 international units of vitamin D per ounce, which is equal on average to about 255 micrograms retinol and 2.25 micrograms vitamin D.

Cheese

When rennet is added to warm acidified milk, the milk proteins coagulate forming a firm curd which is treated in various ways to make cheeses of different kinds. Most of the protein, fat and vitamin A and much of the calcium in the milk remain in the curd, while a large part of the lactose and B-vitamins are lost with the whey as it drains away. Further minor changes in vitamin content occur during ripening and storage. Cheddar cheese consists very roughly of one-third protein, one-third fat and one-third water; although methods of preparation differ, the amounts of protein, fat and carbohydrate in whole milk cheeses are fairly similar. *Cottage cheese* is made from skimmed milk and therefore contains very little fat; *cream cheese* has a high fat content. Hard cheeses such as Cheddar and Double Gloucester, are in general of higher nutritive value per ounce than soft cheeses such as Camembert because they contain less moisture. Certain cheeses are made from milk other than cows' milk; for example, Roquefort cheese is made from sheep's milk.

The nutrient composition of dairy **ice cream** varies with the amounts of sugar, milk, dried milk, butterfat and cream which it contains; it can make a useful contribution to the daily intake of energy and calcium, particularly for people who have small appetites or who will not drink milk. Non-dairy ice cream contains vegetable fats instead of or as well as milk fat.

Eggs

Importance in the diet

Eggs make a useful contribution to the daily intake of vitamin D, retinol, riboflavin, iron and protein in the average diet and for the elderly they can be a particularly important source of protein, iron, vitamin B_{12} and vitamin D. The extent to which the iron is absorbed is dependent on the other components of the meal; it has been shown for example, that the addition of orange juice increases its absorption.

The shell colour is related to the breed of hen rather than to nutrient content and in this respect it is therefore unimportant; similarly a deep yellow yolk does not necessarily indicate a high vitamin A content since the pigment is not β-carotene.

It has been shown that there is very little practical difference in the composition of eggs obtained from battery, deep litter and free range hens, although free range eggs do contain more vitamin B_{12} than deep litter or battery eggs and more folic acid than battery eggs. There are also small differences in the concentrations of calcium and iron.

Effects of cooking

When eggs are boiled or fried the proteins coagulate first in the white at approximately 60°C (140°F), then in the yolk. This property of coagulation makes eggs suitable for binding dry ingredients together in cooking, and for thickening sauces and soups; the mixture of eggs and milk sets in baked egg custard. Over-cooking causes the proteins to curdle and contract slightly and a yellow watery fluid separates out; this may occur when scrambling eggs or boiling sauces to which eggs have been added.

The black discoloration which is sometimes present around the yolk of hard boiled eggs is iron sulphide which is formed during cooking from hydrogen sulphide in the egg white and iron in the egg yolk; this blackening can be reduced by cooling the eggs in water immediately after cooking. When egg whites are beaten, the proteins will hold air and form a stable foam which coagulates or sets at a very low temperature, as for example in meringues. Eggs are also used as raising agents, e.g., in sponge cakes, and to promote the emulsification of fat, e.g., in mayonnaise. Some of the heat-sensitive B-vitamins are lost during cooking. For example, the average loss of thiamin which results from boiling, frying, poaching and scrambling is between 5 and 15 per cent; similar losses of riboflavin also occur. During frying, the fat content of eggs may be increased by about 50 per cent.

Meat

The average nutrient composition of various types of meat is shown in Appendix 2. Changes in methods of animal husbandry have led to the slaughter of younger animals; the meat is therefore more tender and has less fat than before and its flavour tends to be less pronounced.

Muscle tissue is composed of bundles of muscle fibres surrounded by connective tissue and associated with intramuscular fat. Each separate muscle fibre is a tube composed largely of water, and containing soluble proteins, mineral salts, vitamins and flavours. The eating quality of meat is largely determined by the relative proportions of connective tissue and muscle fibres in a particular joint and the amount of 'marbling' fat that is present within the lean, but the overall nutrient content of the lean meat in the more expensive cuts is not significantly different from that in other parts of the carcase.

Importance in the diet

Meat is a good source of high quality protein, available iron, and B-vitamins; pork, bacon and ham in particular are rich in thiamin. Liver and to a lesser extent kidney, are also rich in vitamin A (thus differing from carcase meat) and in iron, riboflavin and other B-vitamins. Sweetbreads and tripe are useful and easily digestible sources of animal protein. Tripe also contains more calcium than other meats; this is derived from the lime with which it is treated during preparation. Chicken, liver and kidney contain less fat than most carcase meat and their energy content is therefore lower.

Consumption of poultry meat is four times greater than in 1955; this trend is due to the growth of the broiler industry and the consequent fall in the price of poultry. Small differences in the nutrient composition of broiler chickens and free range chickens are of no significance in a mixed diet.

Effects of cooking

The muscle protein myoglobin which provides the red colour of raw meat is changed by heat, and the brown colour associated with cooked meat develops at temperatures above 65°C. Heat causes the proteins in the muscle fibres to coagulate and the meat becomes firm: shrinkage occurs and this in turn causes extrusion of meat juices and a loss of weight. Losses of fat and meat juices increase as the temperature rises, and the total weight loss is influenced by the cooking temperature and the internal temperature to which the meat is cooked. Variations in the proportions of muscle, fat and connective tissue in different parts of the carcase also affect weight loss; the following losses may be used (e.g., with food tables) as a rough guide: frying or grilling chops or steaks, 30 per cent; roasting joints, 25 per cent; and frying or grilling bacon, 50 per cent.

Some cheaper cuts of meat which contain a higher proportion of connective tissue are more palatable if a slow moist method of cooking, such as stewing or braising, is used for their preparation; this allows the collagen in the connective tissue to be converted to gelatin thus making the meat more tender. Pressure cooking is also useful for this purpose.

Cooking does not affect the minerals present in meat but a proportion of those which are soluble pass into the drip or dissolve in the cooking water. Similarly, since the B-vitamins are all water-soluble, varying amounts will be found in the drip, meat juice of stock. Cooking temperatures have relatively little effect on nicotinic acid or riboflavin; thiamin, pyridoxine, folic acid and pantothenic acid are more sensitive to heat, and destruction varies between 30 and 50 per cent. After cooking, there are only small differences in the content of the B-vitamins in fresh and frozen meat. Vitamin A is relatively stable to heat, and is not affected by most cooking procedures although some loss occurs during frying at high temperatures (above 200°C).

Meat extractives are water-soluble substances from meat which include peptides, B-vitamins and mineral salts; they provide, with fat, most of the flavour and aroma of meat and act as a stimulant to appetite and to the secretion of gastric juice.

Stock can be made by boiling meat bones in water. The hot water extracts only a small amount of fat and gelatin from the bone marrow and a small quantity of extractives which provide the flavour. Stock is usually used as a basis for soup and it is the addition of other ingredients, e.g., milk, fat and flour in cream soups, which provides most of the nutritional value of the soup.

Meat products

The meat content of meat products is controlled by certain Regulations (page 125). The important contribution which they make to the nutrient contents of the average household diet is shown on page 60; average consumption per head is now about the same as for carcase meat.

The most usual methods of *heat treatment* before any domestic cooking are smoking and canning, both of which cause some loss of thiamin and a slight reduction in the quality of the meat protein. The loss of thiamin when meat is canned is generally slightly greater than in cooked meat. Corned beef is prepared from cured meat which is trimmed, coarsely cut and cooked before canning; after this process very little thiamin remains in the finished product. Commercial *meat extract* is a by-product of corned beef manufacture. The liquid in which successive batches of meat have been heated is concentrated after the removal of the fat. When the meat extract containing the dissolved solids is diluted again for consumption, the amount of protein and energy which it contributes to the soup or beverage is too small to be of importance in the diet; nevertheless it contains minerals and vitamins and is a useful stimulant to appetite.

There is no evidence of any significant loss of nutrients from meat during *freezing*, but the drip which collects on thawing will contain some soluble nutrients.

Fish

Importance in the diet

The flesh or muscle of fish is a valuable source of protein which is of a similar quality to that of meat and milk. It can be seen from Appendix 2 that the amount of fat in different kinds of fish varies widely; the flesh of white fish, such as cod, haddock, plaice and whiting, contains very little fat (1–2 per cent) while that of fatty fish (herring, trout, salmon, eel) varies from 10 per cent to more than 20 per cent. In general, the vitamin content of white fish muscle is similar to that of lean meat. The fat-soluble vitamins A and D are present in the flesh of fatty fish and in the livers of fish such as cod and halibut; oils from the latter may therefore be used as concentrated vitamin supplements. Fish muscle also contains a well balanced supply of minerals including iodine, and if the bones are eaten, as for example in sardines and canned salmon, these are a good source of calcium and phosphorus.

Effects of cooking and processing

The changes that occur when fish is cooked are similar to those in meat but the shrinkage is not so great; losses of mineral salts are proportional to the loss of water. The vitamin A and vitamin D in fatty fish are both heat stable. When fish is canned or cured by smoking there is some loss of thiamin, but otherwise these processes have little effect on the nutrients in fish. Modern methods of freezing do not affect the nutritive value. For estimating the cooked weight of fish, a loss of about 15 per cent may be assumed on gentle cooking.

Sugars and preserves

White sugar provides energy and no other nutrient. Brown sugars and honey also include insignificant quantities of minerals and some B-vitamins, but nowhere near enough of the latter to assist with the metabolism of the sugars present (page 43). Some preserves contain vitamin C and chocolate contains iron, but the main function of all these foods in the diet is to increase palatability.

Vegetables

Importance in the diet

Notwithstanding the fact that they contain 80–95 per cent of water, vege-tables, including potatoes, supply appreciable quantities of nutrients in

71

the average diet and they are also a major source of dietary fibre (page 7). The low energy content and bulky nature of many vegetables (and fruits) are responsible for their extensive use in the many attractive and appetizing meals which are frequently recommended to 'slimmers' (page 90). The composition of different vegetables is given in Appendix 2; their nutrient content is influenced by a number of factors during growth and after harvesting and different samples of the same vegetable can vary considerably. For example, the amount of vitamin C will vary with variety, maturity and exposure to sunlight, as well as with the method of handling and the temperature during transport.

Green vegetables

These are of nutritional importance because of their contribution to the daily intake of vitamin C, β-carotene (which after absorption is converted to vitamin A in the body), folic acid, iron and other minerals. They are especially valuable when eaten raw, as they will suffer no cooking losses; there will be, however, considerable losses of vitamin C in wilted vegetables.

Potatoes

In many diets potatoes provide the main source of vitamin C, even though the vitamin content per unit weight is comparatively low. The amount is highest in new potatoes and falls gradually during post-harvest storage. Instant potato powder and potato flakes or granules are only nutritionally equivalent alternatives to fresh potatoes if the vitamin C and thiamin which are lost in processing are added back to the products. Because of the comparatively large amounts which are eaten, potatoes contribute more protein and iron than other vegetables in the average diet and they are also useful sources of thiamin and nicotinic acid.

Root vegetables

About one-fifth of the average daily intake of vitamin A is provided by vegetables, most of this (14 per cent) by carrots. In contrast, turnips, swedes and parsnips are comparatively good sources of vitamin C, but they contain no β-carotene.

Peas and beans

Green peas, broad beans, haricot beans and other edible seeds such as soya beans are rich in protein and provide more energy and B-vitamins than green and root vegetables; green garden peas and broad beans (but not canned processed peas, dried peas or baked beans) also contain vitamin C.

It is important to remember that the apparently high levels of nutrients shown in dried peas and beans in Appendix 2 will fall when the vegetables are soaked before use.

Soya flour and other products derived from beans are increasingly being used in manufactured foods. They are nutritionally valuable, and extra nutrients may also be added if they are intended to resemble meat (see page 15).

Effects of cooking

The main purpose of cooking vegetables is to soften the cellular tissue and to gelatinize any starch that may be present so that it can be more easily digested.

Weight changes in preparation and cooking Peeling and trimming may reduce the purchased weight of some vegetables by up to one-third or more (Appendix 2); changes in the weight of most raw vegetables during boiling are small and may be ignored when making calculations from food tables.

Nutrient losses After peeling or shredding, vitamin C is rapidly destroyed by oxidation either directly or by the action of an enzyme present in the plant tissues. This loss can be kept to a minimum by preparing vegetables immediately before use and by plunging them into boiling water at the start of the cooking process, when the enzyme will be destroyed.

During cooking, nutrient losses in vegetables (and to a smaller extent in fruit) are mainly caused by the passage of soluble mineral salts and vitamins from the tissues into the cooking water, and by the destruction of some vitamins by heat. Thus, some vitamin C and thiamin are inevitably lost when water is used for cooking because they are both heat sensitive and water soluble. It follows that the greater the volume of water used, the greater is the loss. Green vegetables, which have a large surface area, lose on the average between 50 and 75 per cent of their vitamin C during cooking. Average losses from potatoes are:

	per cent
Boiled in their skins	20–40
Baked in their skins	20–40
Fried	25–35
Boiled after peeling	30–50

If cooked potatoes are mashed and then kept hot, the loss of vitamin C is greater than if they are left whole under similar conditions.

There is a further loss of vitamin C if there is a delay in service and vegetables are kept hot for any length of time. This appears to be accelerated when sodium bicarbonate has been added to the cooking water. For example, after keeping hot for 30 minutes, cabbage will only contain about 60 per cent of its freshly cooked value, and the amount of vitamin C may fall to 40 per cent after one hour.

Potato whiteners or sulphite dips prevent the discoloration of raw pre-peeled potatoes when they are prepared centrally for distribution to restaurants and other catering establishments, but the amount of thiamin which is lost when the treated potatoes are boiled or fried as chips and subsequently kept hot is greatly increased by this treatment.

Effects of processing

The general effects of processing on the nutritive value of foods are discussed on page 61.

Freezing does not in itself cause losses of vitamins, but during *canning* there is some destruction of those vitamins which are unstable to heat (see page 63).

When sulphite is added to dehydrated vegetables to preserve vitamin C and prevent deterioration of quality during storage most of the thiamin is destroyed. In general, this loss is not serious because in a mixed diet the thiamin is obtained from many foods.

Fruit

Fruit is nutritionally most important as a major source of vitamin C in the diet, but it must be remembered that the amount in different fruits varies widely and will always be rather lower after cooking. Blackcurrants are exceptionally rich, followed by strawberries and other soft fruits, oranges, grapefruit and canned and bottled fruit juices (but not fruit squash). Apples, bananas, cherries and rhubarb are examples of fruits which contain much less of the vitamin and which do not in this respect compare favourably with green vegetables. Vitamin C may be added to some fruit products such as apple juice and rose hip syrup. Most fruits also contain sugars and small amounts of other vitamins and minerals.

Dried fruits such as currants, sultanas, raisins, dates and figs provide energy, principally in the form of sugar. Prunes and dried apricots are also useful sources of β-carotene. Dried fruits do not contain vitamin C.

Nuts are rich in fat and protein and are consequently a concentrated source of energy. They are a good source of the B-vitamins, but contain no vitamins A or C.

Cereals

Importance in the diet

Cereal grains are a major component of man's diet throughout the world. In Britain, wheat in the form of bread, flour, cakes, biscuits and pasta together with other cereals provides more than a quarter of the total energy, protein, carbohydrate and iron in the average household diet; cereals also make a substantial contribution to the intake of many other nutrients, particularly calcium, nicotinic acid and thiamin (page 60). In general, the common cereals (wheat, oats, barley, rye, maize and rice) contain 70–77 per cent carbohydrate (starch), 7–14 per cent protein, 2–7 per cent fat and approximately 12 per cent moisture in the whole grain. Recent advances in plant breeding have led to the development of some new cereal varieties which are richer in lysine; some increases in protein levels may be obtained experimentally by the appropriate use of manures and fertilizers.

Nutrient losses in milling

The distribution of nutrients within the wheat grain is not uniform. The concentration of protein, minerals and vitamins is higher in the germ and outer layers of the grain than in the inner starchy endosperm; thus when wheat is milled to produce white flour a proportion of the nutrients is discarded with the bran and germ. Because of the preference for white flour in the British diet, those nutrients lost in the refining process which are of importance in relation to the whole diet are restored. Similar losses occur in the milling of rice unless it is parboiled.

The composition of flour in the UK is controlled by certain Orders and Regulations (page 126) which at present require that all flours contain the following minimum quantities of two B-vitamins (thiamin and nicotinic acid) and iron which correspond to the levels occurring naturally in 80 per cent extraction flour[1]:

	per 100 g
Iron	1.65 mg
Thiamin (vitamin B_1)	0.24 mg
Nicotinic acid	1.60 mg

White flours of about 73 per cent extraction, as now used, have to be fortified with these nutrients to bring their concentrations to the prescribed levels; wholemeal flours contain more than the specified minimum quantities. In addition calcium carbonate must be added to all flours except

---

[1]The weight of flour obtained from a given weight of grain, expressed as a percentage, is known as the *extraction rate*.

wholemeal and certain self-raising flours at the rate of about 14 oz per 280 lb sack (i.e 235–390 mg/100 g).

Wholemeal and white flours

The composition of both wholemeal and white flours varies, but in general wholemeal flour contains somewhat greater amounts of protein, iron, some other minerals, and several vitamins, particularly of the B group, and less calcium than the flours to which calcium is added. Wholemeal flour also contains more indigestible fibre and phytic acid than white flour. However, nutritional differences between wholemeal and fortified white flours are unlikely to be of practical significance in a mixed diet.

Flours which will produce a large loaf of good quality need to contain 'strong' varieties of wheat; these have a slightly higher protein content than the 'weak' wheats which form the greater proportion of flours suitable for making biscuits and cakes.

Effects of cooking and processing

Cooking causes the starch granules of which cereal carbohydrate is composed to swell and gelatinize, thus making the starch digestible (page 6); it also results in a tripling (approximately) of the weight of rice, spaghetti and macaroni on boiling as they take up water.

Thiamin is the vitamin mainly affected during the baking or processing of cereal products because it is sensitive to heat, and destroyed by alkali. The amount lost therefore varies with the cooking time and the final temperature of the cooked food, and whether or not baking powder is used as for example in bread or scones. Riboflavin and nicotinic acid are more stable to heat and the loss on baking is small.

In bread making the yeast gradually ferments the sugars which are formed from the starch in the dough, breaking them down to alcohol and then to carbon dioxide and water which are driven off, thus causing the bread to rise. When water is added to the flour in the preparation of the dough the proteins gliadin and glutenin combine to form gluten. During baking, the yeast is killed and fermentation ceases. The gluten holds the gas and then coagulates as cooking proceeds, holding the bread in shape. The average loss of thiamin in baking bread is about 15 per cent.

About 80 per cent of the bread sold in Britain is now made by the *Chorleywood Bread Process* in which conventional fermentation of the dough is replaced by a few minutes of intense mechanical agitation in special high speed mixers. Breads produced by this process do not differ significantly in nutritional value from those made by conventional methods.

Toast

When bread is toasted the thiamin content is further reduced; the total loss on toasting varies between 15 per cent in thick slices and 30 per cent in thin slices. The heat drives off water from the bread, so that the content of energy and other nutrients per unit weight increases.

Cakes

When making a cake, such as a Madeira cake, air is introduced into the mixture by creaming together the fat and sugar. The eggs are lightly beaten to incorporate air before adding to the creamed mixture and the flour is folded in lightly so that this air is not forced out. During cooking the starch gelatinizes and the flour and egg proteins coagulate. The loss of thiamin when making cakes and biscuits varies between 20 and 30 per cent.

Breakfast cereals

The heat treatment used in the preparation of breakfast cereals destroys a large proportion of the thiamin present in the whole grain. In puffed and flaked products it is usually a total loss but the process used in the preparation of shredded wheat is less drastic and only about half the thiamin is destroyed. Many breakfast cereals are therefore enriched with vitamin B_1 (thiamin), riboflavin and nicotinic acid; protein, iron, vitamin D and sugar are also added to some products. When porridge is made from coarse oatmeal the cooking loss of thiamin is about 10 per cent.

Alcohol

The alcohol in alcoholic drinks is rapidly absorbed from the digestive tract and utilized as a source of energy, 1 gram of alcohol providing

Table 25. **Energy constituents of some alcoholic drinks, per 100 ml**

	Alcohol	Carbohydrate	Energy	
	g	g	kcal	kJ
Brown ale, bottled	2.2	3.0	28	117
Beer, keg bitter	3.0	2.3	31	129
Stout, bottled	2.9	4.2	37	156
Cider, sweet	3.7	4.3	42	176
Sherry, sweet	15.6	6.9	136	568
White wine, dry	9.1	0.6	66	275
White wine, sweet	10.2	5.9	94	394
Red wine	9.5	0.3	68	284
Spirits 70° proof	31.7	0	222	919

7 kilocalories or 29 kilojoules. The alcoholic strength of wines and spirits is shown in this country by a *proof* measure, 100 degrees proof spirit being equivalent to about 49 per cent alcohol by weight or 57 per cent by volume. Carbohydrate may also be present in varying proportions and this provides additional energy. Consumption of spirits, beer and wine continues to rise and it is estimated that in the UK more than 200 kcal (850 kJ) per adult per day are on average obtained from alcoholic drink.

Chronic alcoholics may obtain a large proportion of their energy intake from alcohol and eat very little food. Beer contains significant amounts of riboflavin and nicotinic acid, but spirits contain no vitamins; inevitably the displacement of food by alcohol leads to a marked reduction in the intake of protein, vitamins and many other nutrients.

12 Nutritional value of meals

Number of meals per day

A meal can be arbitrarily defined as the amount of food eaten at one period of time, and which provides 200 kcal (850 kJ) or more. This definition covers much more than the popular meaning of the word, which is that of hot, cooked food eaten while sitting down. People may eat from two to six meals a day, the arrangement being determined mainly by custom and by working conditions and the time taken to travel to and from work. Although the amounts of nutrients in different meals may vary, the total intake of each nutrient must meet an individual's needs, ideally each day and certainly over a period of a week, if the food eaten is to be fully adequate for health.

There is evidence that the number of meals taken in a day (and consequently the amount of food eaten at one time) influences the pattern of utilization of nutrients by the body.

Breakfast

Because of the length of time since the previous meal, and the lower efficiency of the muscles in the morning, it is good nutritional practice to eat breakfast before starting work. It is particularly important for children

Light breakfast	Energy kcal	Protein g	Cooked breakfast	Energy kcal	Protein g
Breakfast cereal (1 oz)	104	2.4	Bacon, one rasher		
Sugar (¼ oz)	28	0	(1 oz)	120	4.1
Milk (4 oz)	72	3.6	Egg (2 oz)	84	7.0
Toast (1 large slice			Toast (2 oz bread)	132	4.4
bread 2 oz)	132	4.4	Butter (¼ oz)	52	0
Butter (¼ oz)	52	0	Marmalade (½ oz)	37	0
Marmalade (½ oz)	37	0	Milk in tea (2 oz)	36	1.8
Milk in tea (2 oz)	36	1.8			
Total	461	12.2	Total	461	17.3

to have a good breakfast before school because this helps to keep them alert during the morning. A quick meal consisting of breakfast cereal with a generous amount of milk and a sprinkling of sugar, followed by toast and marmalade and tea provides the same amount of energy but less protein then a traditional cooked breakfast of bacon and egg (page 79).

If coffee made with milk is substituted for tea in the light breakfast the difference in the protein content is for practical purposes negligible. Both meals would benefit by the addition of some fruit or fruit juice rich in vitamin C.

Eating between meals

If children eat sweets or chocolates between meals, they are likely to have a reduced appetite for vegetables, cereals or meat at the next main meal. This is bad nutritional practice. Firstly, the intake of protein and other nutrients from the main meal will be reduced, and secondly, excessive consumption of sweets can result in severe dental decay. Eating high energy foods between meals, particularly those rich in fat or sugar (such as crisps and chocolate biscuits), can also result in an undesirable increase in weight if the total daily energy intake then exceeds the energy used up. For adults, alcoholic drinks are frequently a cause of excess energy intake.

Calculation of nutrients in prepared dishes and meals using food tables

Dishes

Appendix 2 gives the nutrient composition of foodstuffs per 100 g and per ounce. Knowing the recipe, the approximate nutritional value of a dish containing several ingredients can be worked out by arithmetic. To illustrate this, the calculation of the nutritional value of a bread and butter pudding is shown in Table 26. In this example allowance has been made for the change in weight which occurs during cooking.

Meals

It is quite common to find, particularly in canteens, two types of meals being served: one the sandwich type, the other a cooked meal. The first, for example, could be two cheese and tomato sandwiches and coffee, which many people might not consider to be a meal at all. The second could be roast lamb, peas and chips, followed by canned peaches and custard. The nutritional value of these two meals has been calculated in Table 27 from the figures given in Appendix 2. These calculations show that the meals are of roughly equal energy value, but that the snack

Table 26. **Nutrients in bread and butter pudding**

Ingredient	Weight	Energy		Protein	Fat	Carbo-hydrate	Cal-cium	Iron	Vitamin A (retinol equiva-lent)	Thia-min	Ribo-flavin	Nico-tinic acid equiva-lent	Vitamin C	Vitamin D
	g	kcal	kJ	g	g	g	mg	mg	µg	mg	mg	mg	mg	µg
Bread, white	75	175	743	5.9	1.3	37.3	75	1.3	0	0.14	0.02	1.7	0	0
Butter	20	148	608	0.1	16.4	0	3	0	197	0	0	0	0	0.15
Milk	500	325	1,360	16.5	19.0	23.5	600	0.5	195	0.20	0.95	4.5	10.0	0.10
Sugar	30	118	504	0	0	31.5	1	0	0	0	0	0	0	0
Eggs (2)	100	147	612	12.3	10.9	0	52	2.0	140	0.09	0.47	3.7	0	1.75
Sultanas	50	125	533	0.9	0	32.4	26	0.9	3	0.05	0.04	0.3	0	0
Whole pudding	675[1]	1,038	4,360	35.7	47.6	124.7	757	4.7	535	0.48	1.48	10.2	10.0	2.00
Composition:														
per 100 g		154	649	5.3	7.1	18.5	112	0.7	79	0.06[2]	0.22	1.5	1.5	0.30
per ounce		44	184	1.5	2.0	5.2	32	0.2	23	0.02[2]	0.06	0.4	0.4	0.08

[1] The total weight will not be the same as the sum of the ingredients owing to the loss of moisture on cooking.
[2] 15 per cent deducted to allow for loss in cooking.

81

Table 27. Comparison of the nutritional value of a snack and a cooked meal

	Weight	Energy	Protein	Fat	Carbo-hydrate	Cal-cium	Iron	Vitamin A (retinol equivalent)	Thiamin	Ribo-flavin	Nicotinic acid equivalent	Vitamin C	Vitamin D
	oz	kcal	g	g	g	mg	mg	µg	mg	mg	mg	mg	µg
Snack meal													
Bread, white	4.0	264.0	8.80	2.00	56.40	112.0	2.00	0	0.200	0.040	2.40	0	0
Butter	0.5	105.0	0.05	11.60	0	2.0	0	139.5	0	0	0	0	0.110
Cheese	2.0	230.0	14.80	19.00	0	454.0	0.20	234.0	0.020	0.280	3.60	0	0.140
Lettuce	0.5	1.5	0.15	0	0.15	3.0	0.15	23.5	0.010	0.010	0.05	2.00	0
Tomato	1.0	4.0	0.20	0	0.80	4.0	0.10	28.0	0.020	0.010	0.20	6.00	0
Coffee, instant	0.1	2.8	0.41	0	0.31	4.5	0.12	0	0	0.003	0.71	0	0
Milk (summer)	2.0	36.0	1.80	2.20	2.60	68.0	0	26.0	0.020	0.100	0.60	0.80	0.060
Total		643.3	26.21	34.80	60.26	647.5	2.57	451.0	0.270	0.443	7.56	8.80	0.310
Cooked meal													
Lamb, roast	2.5	207.5	16.25	15.75	0	5.0	1.50	0	0.050	0.175	6.50	0	0
Peas, boiled	2.0	24.0	3.00	0.20	2.40	18.0	0.80	28.0	0.140	0.040	1.40	8.0	0
Chips, fried	3.0	216.0	3.30	9.30	31.80	12.0	0.60	0	0.090	0.030	1.80	12.0	0
Peaches, canned	4.0	100.0	0.40	0	26.00	4.0	0.40	48.0	0	0.040	0.80	4.0	0
Custard	3.0	99.0	3.30	3.60	14.40	120.0	0	36.0	0.030	0.180	0.90	0	0.030
Total		646.5	26.25	28.85	74.60	159.0	3.30	112.0	0.310	0.465	11.40	24.0	0.030

For simplicity weights of food are given only in ounces (28.35 g = 1 oz) meal is in some respects of higher nutritional value than the hot meal. Thus it provides the same amount of protein, four times as much vitamin A and calcium, but less of some other nutrients.

The vitamin C content of the cooked meal is substantially higher, but if the sandwiches had been accompanied by an orange or some watercress, there is little to choose in terms of nutrient content between the two meals. A cold or 'packed' meal is thus not necessarily inferior to a 'cooked' meal: its nutritional value depends on the quantities and nutritional composition of the items in it.

Allowance for waste

The calculation of the nutritional value of a meal or a diet *as actually eaten* cannot be made directly from the total amounts of the foods bought from the shops, nor from the total food used in the kitchen. There is always a proportion of waste for which allowance must be made, that is:

1. INEDIBLE WASTE, e.g. egg shells, potato peelings, outer leaves of cabbages, orange peel, bacon rinds, bones and gristle of meat etc.
2. EDIBLE WASTE
    (a) *Preparation losses,* e.g., batter left in mixing bowls, fat left in frying pans, crusts from bread, spilt milk.
    (b) *Table waste,* e.g., scraps left on plates.
    (c) *Pet food,* e.g., edible scraps fed to domestic pets, garden birds, ducks.
    (d) Edible food which has 'gone bad' and is discarded.

Inedible waste

Average figures for the inedible waste associated with different foods are given in Appendix 2, as a percentage of the purchased weight. If, for example, you buy a pound of bananas (item 88), 40 per cent is inedible waste, which in this case is the skin.

The food tables give the nutrients in the 'edible portion' only, and if they are used for calculating the nutritional value of foods where only the purchased weight is known, the percentage of inedible waste must be deducted. For example, the energy value of one pound of bananas (purchased weight) is $16 \times \dfrac{100-40}{100} \times$ kcal per ounce (from Table 2, Appendix 2)

$$= \frac{16 \times 60 \times 22}{100}$$

$$= 211 \text{ kcal}$$

Further examples of this type of calculation are given in Appendix 3.

The percentage of inedible waste in a food varies with the exact nature of the food and with quality. For example it varies between different cuts of lamb or different sizes and varieties of orange.

Edible waste

It is often difficult for practical reasons to measure the amount of food actually eaten. An allowance for loss of edible food must then be made before the nutritional adequacy of any diet is worked out. The average wastage in cooking, on plates, and from food given to pets, has usually been assumed to be 10 per cent, but of course the amount varies from food to food and from family to family.

Planning balanced meals and nutritionally adequate diets

The provision of palatable and acceptable meals is the first consideration; only then can planning for good nutrition be effective.

A *balanced meal* is one which provides adequate amounts of proteins and all the minerals and vitamins as well as energy. The main sources of each nutrient are discussed in Chapters 2–8. The *total daily intake* of each major nutrient which is recommended for groups of people of different ages and occupations is given on page 54, and these figures may be used as targets at which to aim when planning a diet.

The food composition tables in Appendix 2 show that nearly all foods contain several nutrients and that most minerals and vitamins are present in a large number of foods in common use. Thus the simplest way to meet these nutritional standards is to eat a varied diet, containing a wide selection of foods. The amount of food eaten is to a large extent limited by its energy content because appetite usually controls food intake to satisfy energy needs.

Experience and custom have influenced food choice in such a way that traditional British meals are generally nutritionally satisfactory as well as good to eat; nevertheless to be sure that this is achieved, now that we rely to a greater extent on snacks and convenience foods, certain general rules can be followed:

(a) Each meal should contain some foods rich in *protein*, such as meat, poultry, fish, cheese, eggs, milk, bread and flour, nuts, peas and beans.

(b) Each main meal should contain plenty of *fruit* and *vegetables*, which are good sources of some vitamins and minerals.

(c) Foods rich in energy should be eaten in amounts which will satisfy appetite and maintain correct body weight. These include butter and margarine (which also provide vitamins A and D), bread (which also provides protein, minerals and vitamins), and only then jam, cakes and biscuits, sugary foods and other foods rich in fat and carbohydrate.

Planning meals in relation to cost

Within this general framework it is usually necessary to consider the relative cost of different sources of nutrients. Allowance must also be made for the effects of cooking on nutritive value (see page 62).

Great savings in the cost of eating can be made with a thorough knowledge of food composition and nutritional value for money. For example, cheaper cuts of meat have practically the same nutritional value as the more expensive cuts although they may take longer to cook. Many meat

Table 28. Cheap sources of energy and nutrients (In approximate[1] order of cheapness, the cheapest being first)

Energy	Sugar, lard, margarine, butter, white bread, old potatoes, brown bread, biscuits, breakfast cereals.
Protein	White bread, brown bread, milk, cheese, old potatoes, baked beans, chicken, eggs, breakfast cereals, liver, fish.
Carbohydrate	Sugar, white bread, old potatoes, brown bread, breakfast cereals, new potatoes, biscuits.
Calcium	Milk, cheese, white bread, ice cream, brown bread, carrots.
Iron	Liver, canned beans, old potatoes, brown bread, white bread, breakfast cereals, frozen peas, fresh green vegetables.
Vitamin A	Carrots, liver, margarine, butter, cheese, milk.
Thiamin	Fortified breakfast cereals, potatoes, bread, frozen peas, milk, pork.
Riboflavin	Liver, fortified breakfast cereals, milk, eggs, ice cream, cheese, potatoes.
Nicotinic acid	Fortified breakfast cereals, potatoes, liver, white bread, chicken, brown bread, milk, frozen peas.
Vitamin C	Fruit juices, oranges, new potatoes, fresh green vegetables, tomatoes, frozen peas.
Vitamin D	Margarine, fatty fish, butter, eggs.

When harvests are badly affected by weather conditions, the nutritional value for money provided by some of these foods may decline.

products also provide good nutritional value for money. Again, cheaper fatty fish such as herring or mackerel has the same nutritional value as expensive fatty fish such as salmon. The cheaper fresh vegetables such as cabbage, carrots and potatoes are often much better value for money than many canned or frozen vegetables. Fresh citrus fruits are very convenient sources of vitamin C and are also fairly cheap. Cheese and eggs can take the place of meat in a main course.

Section 3 of Appendix 3 shows how the amounts of protein, vitamins or any nutrients bought for one penny can be calculated for any food by using the food composition tables and the price of the food. The precise relationship between foods will vary according to the time of year and current prices, but Table 28 gives general idea of some *cheap* sources of certain nutrients. It is important to realize that a cheap source of one nutrient may not be a cheap food in the context of the whole diet, as with sugar where only one nutrient is supplied. Bread, milk, cheese, offals, potatoes, peas and beans, and breakfast cereals, on the other hand, supply several nutrients cheaply and are thus very good value for money.

Planning meals for the week ahead is most important in food budgeting. Careful shopping, correct preparation and storage of food, and a good standard of cookery all play a part in using the available money to the best advantage.

13 Needs of special groups of people

Infants and young children

Infants are unique in that they must rely on a single food, milk, to satisfy all their nutritional needs. Breast milk is ideal for several reasons:
  (a) All the nutrients are present in the right amount for human infants, and in a readily absorbed form. Those nutrients which are low, such as iron and copper, are those which are already stored in large amounts in the infant's liver.
  (b) It contains several natural agents which protect against disease.
  (c) It is clean, cannot be prepared incorrectly, and does not cause allergies.
A mother should therefore try to breast feed her baby for at least 2 weeks, and ideally for 4–6 months. Few mothers are unable to breast feed. Some cannot for medical reasons, but more prefer not to do so and use cows' milk, which has been modified to some extent so that it is more like human milk. Because the immature kidney of the young infant is unable to adapt to the higher concentrations of protein and some minerals in cows' milk it is very important to make up these feeds exactly according to the instructions so that they are not overconcentrated.

Solid foods should not be introduced before 4 months of age. There is no advantage to the baby to do so and there may be some risks of developing allergies and of becoming obese. From about 6 months onwards the mother may gradually introduce infant cereal foods, pureed fruit and vegetables, egg yolk, and even finely divided meat (using little or preferably no salt or sugar). By about 12–18 months, the infant can eat a mixed diet not very different from that of the rest of the family. Milk will continue to be very important but less will be drunk as more solid foods are eaten.

Schoolchildren

Schoolchildren are growing fast and are also very active. Table 22 on page 54 gives the recommended intakes of energy and nutrients for groups of children of different ages and shows that these are high in relation to their body size compared with those of adults. For example, the requirements of 9–12 year old girls for energy, protein, calcium and some other nutrients are higher than those of grown women in most occupations. The big appetites of children usually reflect a real nutritional need rather than greed. Because of their smaller size compared with adults, and correspondingly small stomachs, it is important that children should eat meals which are not too bulky. Bread, milk, cheese, meat, fish, liver, eggs, fruit and green vegetables and potatoes are excellent sources of a number of nutrients. Milk is one of the best sources of calcium, riboflavin and protein. Children should be taught sensible eating habits from an early age: biscuits, sweets, soft drinks, chips and crisps should not be allowed to displace other more useful foods too often.

Adolescents

The nutrient needs of adolescents are higher in many respects than those of any other group. Healthy adolescents have very big appetites and it is important that they should satisfy them with food of high nutritional value in the form of well balanced meals (page 84) rather than by too many high energy snacks. Obesity among schoolchildren is nowadays probably one of the commonest forms of malnutrition and this may continue into adult life. There is some evidence that adolescent obesity may be partly due to a general decrease in physical activity and hence in energy expenditure rather than to an excessive energy intake. A knowledge of nutrition and the incentive to apply this knowledge in practice is likely to benefit the health of young people for the rest of their lives. Dental decay is very common in British schoolchildren; sweet and sticky foods and snacks eaten between meals are one cause of this (page 8).

School meals

Under the Provision of Milk and Meals Regulations, 1969 (under review), made by the Secretary of State for Education and Science, school dinners should be provided which are suitable in all respects as the main meal of the day; they can include not only set dinners but also a selection of à la carte dishes.

The nutritional standards were the subject of a report *Nutrition in Schools* (Report of the Working Party on the Nutritional Aspects of School Meals, Department of Education and Science, HMSO, 1975) which recommends that the edible portion of the food bought for the school meal should provide, on average, 880 kcal (3.68 MJ) and 29 g protein. Some losses of edible food during preparation, cooking and serving are inevitable, but the school dinner *on the plate* should provide the pupils with at least one-third of their recommended daily intake of energy and between one-third and one-half of their recommended intake of protein. Furthermore, menus should be selected and care taken during meal preparation to ensure that adequate amounts of minerals and vitamins are also supplied. The differing requirements of individuals are best met by adjusting the size of their helpings to their appetite.

Pregnancy and Lactation

A woman's nutritional needs increase during pregnancy and lactation (page 54). This is not only because her diet must provide for the growth and development of her child (as below), but other physiological changes occur which ensure that sufficient nutrients are available for the child such as the laying down of new tissues in the woman's own body. Much of the weight gain during the early part of pregnancy is due to the accumulation of fat which provides an energy store to meet the additional demands of the growing fetus and the breast-fed infant.

Approximate weight of an infant at various ages	
Conception	0 kg
4½ months pregnancy	0.5 kg
9 months pregnancy (birth)	3.5 kg
4½ months after birth	7.5 kg

It is most important that the mother's diet contains sufficient energy, protein, iron, calcium, folic acid and vitamins C and D (and liquid during lactation) for building the baby's muscular tissues, bones and teeth, and for the formation of haemoglobin; if it does not, her own stores of nutrients may be reduced. Some good sources of these nutrients are given in Part 1. In practice most of these extra nutrients will be obtained simply by satisfying the appetite with a good mixed diet including plenty of milk, cheese, liver, bread, fruit and vegetables, but special supplements of iron and folic acid are often recommended during pregnancy. A good knowledge of nutrition is invaluable at this stage and will also help the mother to teach sound eating habits to her child in due course.

Old people

There is very little difference between the nutritional requirements of the elderly and the younger adult (page 54), but because the elderly tend to be less active after the age of 75, their average energy requirements are presumed to be slightly less (by 150–200 kilocalories per head per day) and, for some, dietary adjustments such as a reduction in fat consumption will be necessary to avoid an increase in weight. Those with physical disabilities or poor appetites who live alone should be encouraged to cook a mid-day dinner of good nutritional quality and to supplement this with foods such as milk, breakfast cereals, eggs, cheese, bread, and fruits rich in vitamin C, which need little preparation. For the housebound who do not have the benefit of sunlight a good dietary source of vitamin D such as margarine, eggs, fatty fish (e.g., sardines, kippers) or butter is important. Foods rich in fibre may also be beneficial.

Slimmers

Energy needs and food consumption have been discussed in Chapter 5.

Planning a slimming diet is a matter of individual preference. Essentially, the energy intake should be cut down by about 1,000 kilocalories (4 MJ) each day while other nutrients should still reach recommended levels. It is often convenient to cut out sugar and sugary foods such as sweets, preserves, soft drinks, biscuits and puddings as well as alcohol as these are mainly sources of energy rather than nutrients. A 'low carbohydrate diet' works on this principle. Effective slimming diets are all basically 'low calorie diets' (i.e., low energy diets) though they vary in how this is achieved. A good plan is to base meals on a modest helping of lean meat, fish, eggs or cheese with liberal amounts of fruits and vegetables and small amounts of bread and potatoes. Eating three or four meals a day gives better results than eating the same amount of food at one or two meals only; breakfast should be included. As it may take several months to reach the desired weight, a slimming diet should be sensible and palatable enough to be tolerated for this length of time. After this, a diet of reduced energy content may still be needed to maintain the correct weight. Cranky diets based on one or two foods only are rarely successful as they are unrealistic, dull, and some-times expensive; they can also be nutritionally dangerous.

It can be very difficult to reduce food intake. Some people for example turn to food for comfort and others must attend social functions where dieting is difficult. Keeping to a diet can sometimes be made easier by join-ing a slimmers' group.

Vegetarians

Vegetarians do not, for a variety of reasons, eat flesh foods in any form, but the majority consume some animal products, the most important of which are milk, cheese and eggs. Such diets may be rather bulky and lower in energy than a mixed diet because most vegetables have a high water content but, in general, their nutritional value is very similar.

A much smaller group, *vegans*, eat no foods of animal origin at all. Man's nutrient requirements with the exception of vitamin B_{12} (page 47) can be met by a diet composed entirely of plant foods but to do so it must be carefully planned using a wide selection of foods. A mixture of plant proteins derived from cereals, legumes, peas, beans and nuts will provide sufficient protein of good quality, but special care is needed to ensure that sufficient energy, calcium, iron, riboflavin, vitamin B_{12} and vitamin D are also available. Yeast extract is a good source of some of the B-vitamins including vitamin B_{12} which are otherwise found mainly in animal foods.

World food shortages and increasing costs have stimulated interest in the advantages, in terms of food production, of reducing consumption of animal products and of replacing some meat protein by texturized vegetable proteins (page 15) suitably fortified with the nutrients associated with lean meat. This enables familiar food patterns to be maintained.

Organic and Health Foods

All foods, being derived from plants or animals, are organic; and all foods, because they provide nutrients, are conducive to health when eaten as part of a balanced diet as described in this Manual. The words have, however, recently acquired the restricted meaning of foods grown without the use of inorganic fertilizers, pesticides or herbicides, and either not processed or processed without the use of additives. These substances must be used if enough food for our dense urban population is to be grown and distributed economically, and their use is controlled by legislation (page 124). Furthermore, they have little effect on nutritional value, which is largely determined by the species of plant or animal.

People who choose to restrict their diet to such foods should, like vegetarians or anyone else whose diet is limited, take extra care to ensure that they obtain enough of all the nutrients. In extreme cases, such as zen macrobiotic diets where little but whole grain cereals are eaten, intakes of calcium, iron, vitamin B_{12} and vitamin C are likely to be too low for health.

Immigrants

Immigrant communities in Britain which retain their traditional diets and customs may have special dietary problems. In particular, Asian groups may have very low intakes of vitamin D. Because exposure to sunlight (especially by women and children) may also be low due to customs of dress and because they tend to remain indoors, rickets sometimes develops. Good Sources of vitamin D (page 51) should, therefore, be included in sufficient quantity in the diet. The iron content of their traditional diet is also low.

Special diets

The principles set out in this book hold in general for all healthy individuals. There are, however, a few people who possess personal idiosyncracies causing reactions to certain foods, for example, eggs, shellfish or strawberries. In conditions such as diabetes, coeliac disease or lactose intolerance, a special diet should be followed, and, when certain drugs are taken, the avoidance of some foods such as cheese is necessary. These allergies and illnesses are a medical rather than a nutritional problem.

Conclusion: assessing the adequacy of a diet

It is important not only that all the essential nutrients should be present in the foods eaten, but also that they should be present in the amounts required by different people. To find out whether a particular diet is nutritionally adequate, three things must be known:

(a) What foods were eaten?

(b) How much of each food was eaten?

(c) What kind of person or people ate the foods? Were they men, women, adolescents, or children, and were they very active or sedentary? Were any of the women pregnant or nursing a baby?

When the answers to these questions are known, daily nutrient intakes can then be compared with the amounts recommended for health (page 54). It must however be emphasized that the recommendations are high enough to cover the needs of practically all healthy people; therefore it is only when an individual is consistently obtaining less than this recommended intake that there could be cause for concern.

Two important methods of measuring food consumption are:

(a) Measuring the amount of food purchased by, for example, a a family during one week. When the amount of food bought is recorded, it is important to follow up by finding out how much of it is eaten, how much goes into or out of the store cupboard or freezer, how many people ate it, and how much is wasted in preparing meals and on the plate (page 83).

(b) Weighing the foods eaten by an individual at each separate meal (usually for one week). This is the most precise method of assessing the value of a diet; each item of food must be weighed and recorded and any plate waste deducted.

For meals served by canteens or restaurants it is possible to weigh all the components of a number of meals when ready for serving. An estimate of the amounts of nutrients wasted in preparation can be obtained by comparing the calculated nutritional value of the meals served with the calculated nutritional value of the supplies of food entering the kitchen.

As an example of what to do when looking at any meal pattern, the diet of a woman doing normal work has been examined in the following way:

(a) The information on food consumption is first set out in the form of a typical daily menu (Table 29);

(b) The nutrients obtained from each meal are next calculated using food tables, the results being summarized as in Table 30. This shows at a glance the contribution of each meal to the total energy and nutrient intake;

(c) With an understanding of nutrition it is then possible to assess the importance of any differences between nutrient intake and the amounts recommended for health on page 54. In this instance, it can be seen that:

(1) *Energy:* Moderately active women need on average 2,200 kilocalories a day, so that the energy value of the food eaten is a little more than recommended; 44 per cent of the calories come from fat and 41 per cent from carbohydrate.

(2) *Protein:* Women are recommended to obtain 55 grams protein a day; the amount is 1½ times greater than this. In this menu, meat and eggs provide 46 grams protein; bread and potatoes 13 grams.

(3) *Calcium:* The calcium is twice the recommended amount.

(4) *Iron:* The recommended intake for women is 12 mg daily. The total dietary intake is only 10 mg; this is partly because pork contains less iron than some other meats (see Appendix 2). Liver and kidney are particularly rich sources of available iron.

(5) *Vitamin A:* The total intake is four times greater than the recommended intake; if carrots had not been included in the menu the amount would still have been slightly higher than the recommended intake.

(6) The amounts of the B-vitamins (thiamin, riboflavin and nicotinic acid) are roughly double the recommended intakes.

93

(7) *Vitamin C:* After allowing for cooking losses the total of 91 mg is three times greater than the recommended intake. Of this, 40 mg is provided by the orange juice.

(8) *Vitamin D:* This is sufficient. Any dietary source will be supplemented by adequate exposure to sunlight.

Thus this diet is more than adequate in all nutrients except iron but its total energy value and particularly the proportion of calories from fat is rather high.

Table 29. **Menu for one day for a woman doing normal work**

Breakfast		Snack	
Orange juice	4 oz	1 cup of coffee[1]	
Cornflakes	½ oz	Milk	2 oz
Milk	4 oz		
Sugar	¼ oz	**Tea**	
Toast	2 oz	Bread	1 oz
Butter	¼ oz	Butter	⅛ oz
Marmalade	½ oz	Jam	½ oz
2 cups of tea[1]		Biscuits, sweet (2)	½ oz
Milk	2 oz	2 cups of tea[1]	
		Milk	2 oz
Lunch		**Supper**	
Eggs (2) scrambled	4 oz	Pork chop, grilled	4 oz
Margarine	½ oz	Apple sauce:	
Milk	2 oz	Apple	4 oz
Toast	2 oz	Margarine	⅕ oz
Butter	¼ oz	Sugar	¼ oz
Banana	4 oz	Potatoes, boiled	6 oz
Single cream	2 oz	Carrots	4 oz
1 cup of coffee[1]		Ice cream	2 oz
Milk	2 oz	1 cup of coffee[1]	
		Milk	2 oz

[1]The amount of tea or coffee used varies considerably. These arbitrary figures have been used per cup: tea ⅙oz, coffee ¹⁄₁₀oz.

Table 30. **Nutrient content of a menu for a woman doing normal work (See Table 29)**

Meal	Energy		Protein	Fat	Carbo-hydrate	Cal-cium	Iron	Vitamin A (retinol equivalent)	Thia-min	Ribo-flavin	Nicotinic acid equivalent	Vitamin C	Vitamin D
	kcal	kJ	g	g	g	mg	mg	µg	mg	mg	mg	mg	µg
Breakfast	462	1,903	11.4	13.6	75.0	278	1.6	145	0.49	0.56	6.9	43.9	0.18
Snack	39	166	2.2	2.2	2.9	72	0.1	22	0.02	0.10	1.3	0.8	0.04
Lunch	729	3,049	25.0	46.1	57.5	310	4.2	525	0.28	0.88	8.7	13.6	3.34
Tea	232	979	5.0	8.9	35.3	112	0.9	57	0.09	0.12	2.0	2.3	0.07
Supper	786	3,332	40.2	38.6	76.6	221	3.3	2,349	1.04	0.58	16.9	30.8	0.49
Total dietary intake	2,248	9,429 (9.4 MJ)	83.8	109.4	247.3	993	10.1	3,098	1.92	2.24	35.8	91.4	4.12
Recommended intake (1969)	2,200	9.2 MJ	55.0	—	—	500	12.0	750	0.90	1.30	15.0	30.0	2.50

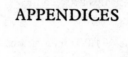

APPENDICES

1 Common measures and conversion factors

Many foods are measured in pounds, ounces and pints, while scientists prefer metric units (grams, millilitres). Energy was measured in *calories*, but the SI units *joules* are increasingly being used. The conversion factors below show the relationships between these.

WEIGHT

1 milligram (mg)	= 1,000 micrograms (μg)	
1 gram (g)	= 1,000 mg	= 0.035 ounces (oz)
1 kilogram (kg)	= 1,000 g	= 2.20 pounds (lb)
1 oz	= 28.35 g	
1 lb	= 453.6 g	

VOLUME

1 litre	= 1,000 millilitres (ml)	= 1.76 pints (pt)
1 pt	= 20 fluid oz	= 568 ml

LENGTH

1 metre (m)	= 100 centimetres (cm)	= 1,000 millimetres (mm)
		= 39.4 inches (in)
1 in	= 2.54 cm	
1 foot (ft)	= 0.3048 m	

ENERGY

1 kilojoule (kJ)	= 1,000 joules (J)	
1 megajoule (MJ)	= 1,000 kJ	= 239 kilocalories (kcal)
1 kcal	= 4.184 kJ	

2 Composition of food

The composition of food is given in two tables:

Table 1: Composition per 100 grams of edible material

Table 2: Composition per ounce of edible material

Average values are given for *raw food unless otherwise stated*. The tables are based chiefly on the 4th revised edition of McCance and Widdowson's *The Composition of Foods* (published by HMSO in 1978) and do not attempt to be comprehensive. For calculating the nutritive value of cooked foods where values are given only for the raw food in the tables, the weight of raw food must be estimated and allowance made for nutrient losses (see Chapters 10 and 11). Allowance must also be made for foods weighed with inedible matter (page 83). The wastage values predict the amount of inedible material in the item as listed; thus for raw lamb it is the percentage of the raw meat which is bone, while for roast lamb it is the proportion of bone in the whole *cooked* product and does not include any fat which may have been lost during roasting. Appendix 3 provides examples of the use of these Tables.

Two of the vitamins are given in the tables in the form of equivalents; these are vitamin A (as retinol equivalents, page 42) and nicotinic acid equivalents (which include the contribution of tryptophan, page 46). The two vitamins are thus expressed in the same form as in the *Recommended Daily Amounts of Food Energy and Nutrients for Groups of People in the United Kingdom* of the Department of Health and Social Security (page 54). Carbohydrate is given as total monosaccharide (page 8).

In Tables 1 and 2 the energy value of the foods is given in kilojoules (kJ) as well as kilocalories; kilojoules are calculated from the protein, fat and carbohydrate content (page 23), and the nutrient values per ounce shown in Table 2 are calculated from those in Table 1.

Table 1. **Composition per 100 g (raw edible weight except where stated)**

No.	Food	Inedible waste	Energy		Protein	Fat	Carbo-hydrate (as mono-saccharide)
		%	kcal	kJ	g	g	g
	Milk						
1	Cream, double	0	447	1,841	1.5	48.2	2.0
2	Cream, single	0	195	806	2.4	19.3	3.2
3	Milk, liquid, whole	0	65	272	3.3	3.8	4.7
4	Milk, condensed, whole sweetened	0	322	1,362	8.3	9.0	55.5
5	Milk, whole, evaporated	0	158	660	8.6	9.0	11.3
6	Milk, UHT	0	65	274	3.3	3.8	4.7
7	Milk, dried, skimmed	0	355	1,512	36.4	1.3	52.8
8	Yogurt, low fat, natural	0	52	216	5.0	1.0	6.2
9	Yogurt, low fat, fruit	0	95	405	4.8	1.0	17.9
	Cheese						
10	Cheese, Cheddar	0	406	1,682	26.0	33.5	0
11	Cheese, cottage	0	96	402	13.6	4.0	1.4
	Meat						
12	Bacon, rashers, raw	11	422	1,744	14.4	40.5	0
13	Bacon, rashers, cooked	0	447	1,851	24.5	38.8	0
14	Beef, average, raw	17	266	1,107	17.1	22.0	0
15	Beef, corned	0	217	905	26.9	12.1	0
16	Beef, stewing steak, raw	3	176	736	20.2	10.6	0
17	Beef, stewing steak, cooked	0	223	932	30.9	11.0	0
18	Black pudding	0	305	1,270	12.9	21.9	15.0
19	Chicken, raw	33	230	954	17.6	17.7	0
20	Chicken, roast, light meat	0	142	599	26.5	4.0	0
21	Ham, cooked	0	269	1,119	24.7	18.9	0
22	Kidney, average	12	89	375	16.2	2.7	0
23	Lamb, average, raw	17	335	1,388	15.9	30.2	0
24	Lamb, roast	25	291	1,209	23.0	22.1	0
25	Liver, average, raw	0	162	680	20.7	8.1	2.0
26	Liver, fried	0	243	1,016	24.9	13.6	5.6
27	Luncheon meat	0	313	1,298	12.6	26.9	5.5
28	Pork, average, raw	26	325	1,343	16.0	29.0	0
29	Pork chop, grilled	22	332	1,380	28.5	24.2	0
30	Sausage, pork	0	367	1,520	10.6	32.1	9.5
31	Sausage beef	0	299	1,242	9.6	24.1	11.7
32	Steak and kidney pie, cooked	0	286	1,195	15.2	18.3	14.6
33	Tripe, dressed	0	60	252	9.4	2.5	0

Water g	Calcium mg	Iron mg	Vitamin A (retinol equivalent) µg	Thiamin mg	Riboflavin mg	Nicotinic acid equivlent mg	Vitamin C mg	Vitamin D µg	No.
49	50	0.2	500	0.02	0.08	0.4	1	0.28	1
72	79	0.3	155	0.03	0.12	0.8	1	0.12	2
87	120	0.1	46[1] 32[2]	0.04	0.19	0.9	2	0.03[1] 0.01[2]	3
26	280	0.2	124	0.08	0.48	2.2	2	0.09	4
69	280	0.2	108	0.06	0.51	2.3	1	2.91[3]	5
88	120	0.1	40	0.04	0.19	0.9	0	0.02	6
4	1,190	0.4	0	0.42	1.60	9.7	6	0	7
86	180	0.1	10	0.05	0.26	1.2	0	0.01	8
75	160	0.2	22	0.05	0.23	1.1	2	0.01	9
37	800	0.4	412	0.04	0.50	6.2	0	0.26	10
79	60	0.1	41	0.02	0.19	3.3	0	0.02	11
41	7	1.0	0	0.36	0.14	5.8	0	0	12
32	12	1.4	0	0.40	0.18	9.2	0	0	13
64	8	1.8	0	0.05	0.17	7.3	0	0	14
58	14	2.9	0	0.01	0.23	9.0	0	0	15
69	8	2.1	0	0.06	0.23	8.5	0	0	16
57	15	3.0	0	0.03	0.33	10.2	0	0	17
44	35	20.0	0	0.09	0.07	3.8	0	0	18
65	10	0.7	0	0.08	0.14	9.3	0	0	19
69	9	0.5	0	0.08	0.14	15.3	0	0	20
54	9	1.3	0	0.44	0.15	8.0	0	0	21
79	9	6.0	120	0.39	1.90	10.7	10	0	22
53	7	1.3	0	0.09	0.19	7.4	0	0	23
54	9	2.1	0	0.10	0.25	9.2	0	0	24
69	6	11.4	14,670	0.26	3.10	18.1	16	0.75	25
56	14	8.8	19,010	0.26	4.30	20.4	12	0.38	26
52	15	1.1	0	0.07	0.12	4.5	0	0	27
54	8	0.8	0	0.59	0.16	7.0	0	0	28
46	11	1.2	0	0.66	0.20	11.0	0	0	29
45	41	1.1	0	0.04	0.12	5.7	0	0	30
50	48	1.4	0	0.03	0.13	7.1	0	0	31
49	37	2.8	126	0.14	0.52	6.8	2	0.55	32
88	75	0.5	0	0	0.01	2.1	0	0	33

[1] Summer value [2] Winter value [3] fortified

Composition per 100 g

No.	Food	Inedible waste	Energy		Protein	Fat	Carbo-hydrate (as mono-saccharide)
		%	kcal	kJ	g	g	g
	Fish						
34	White fish, filleted	5	76	322	17.4	0.7	0
35	Cod, fried in batter	0	199	834	19.6	10.3	7.5
36	Fish fingers	0	178	749	12.6	7.5	16.1
37	Herring	37	234	970	16.8	18.5 [5]	0
38	Kipper fillets	2	184	770	19.8	11.7 [5]	0
39	Salmon, canned	6	155	649	20.3	8.2	0
40	Sardines, canned in oil, fish only	7	217	906	23.7	13.6	0
	Eggs						
41	Eggs, fresh	12	147	612	12.3	10.9	0
	Fats						
42	Butter	0	740	3,041	0.4	82.0	0
43	Lard; cooking fat; dripping	0	892	3,667	0	99.1	0
44	Low-fat spread	0	366	1.506	0	40.7	0
45	Margarine, average	0	730	3,000	0.1	81.0	0
46	Oils, cooking and salad	0	899	3,696	0	99.9	0
	Preserves, etc.						
47	Chocolate, milk	0	529	2,214	8.4	30.3	59.4
48	Honey	0	288	1,229	0.4	0	76.4
49	Jam	0	262	1,116	0.5	0	69.2
50	Marmalade	0	261	1,114	0.1	0	69.5
51	Sugar, white	0	394	1,680	0	0	105.0
52	Syrup	0	298	1,269	0.3	0	79.0
	Vegetables						
53	Beans, canned in tomato sauce	0	64	270	5.1	0.5	10.3
54	Beans, broad	75	69	293	7.2	0.5	9.5
55	Beans, haricot, dry	0	271	1,151	21.4	1.6	45.5
56	Beans, runner	14	24	102	2.3	0	3.9
57	Beetroot, boiled	20	44	189	1.8	0	9.9
58	Brussels sprouts, raw	25	26	111	4.0	0	2.7
59	Brussels sprouts, boiled	0	18	75	2.8	0	1.7
60	Cabbage, green, raw	30	22	92	2.8	0	2.8
61	Cabbage, green, boiled	0	15	66	1.7	0	2.3

[5] Fat content varies throughout the year between 10 and 25 per cent.

Water	Calcium	Iron	Vitamin A (retinol equivalent)	Thiamin	Riboflavin	Nicotinic acid equivalent	Vitamin C	Vitamin D	No.
g	mg	mg	μg	mg	mg	mg	mg	μg	
82	16	0.3	0	0.08	0.07	4.9	0	0	34
61	80	0.5	0	0.04	0.10	6.7	0	0	35
64	43	0.7	0	0.09	0.06	3.1	0	0	36
64	33	0.8	45	0	0.18	7.1	0	22.50	37
68	60	1.2	45	0.02	0.30	7.0	0	22.25	38
70	93	1.4	90	0.04	0.18	10.8	0	12.50	39
58	550	2.9	0	0.04	0.36	12.6	0	7.50	40
75	52	2.0	140	0.09	0.47	3.7	0	1.75	41
15	15	0.2	985	0	0	0.1	0	0.76	42
1	1	0.1	0	0	0	0	0	0	43
57	0	0	900 [3]	0	0	0	0	7.94 [3]	44
16	4	0.3	900 [3]	0	0	0.1	0	7.94 [3]	45
0	0	0	0	0	0	0	0	0	46
2	220	1.6	6.6	0.10	0.23	1.6	0	0	47
23	5	0.4	0	0	0.05	0.2	0	0	48
30	18	1.2	2	0	0	0	10	0	49
28	35	0.6	8	0	0	0	10	0	50
0	2	0	0	0	0	0	0	0	51
20	26	1.5	0	0	0	0	0	0	52
74	45	1.4	50	0.07	0.05	1.3	0	0	53
77	30	1.1	22	0.28	0.05	5.0	30	0	54
11	180	6.7	0	0.45	0.13	5.9	0	0	55
89	27	0.8	50	0.05	0.10	1.3	20	0	56
83	30	0.7	0	0.02	0.04	0.4	5	0	57
88	32	0.7	67	0.10	0.15	1.5	87	0	58
92	25	0.5	67	0.06	0.10	0.9	41	0	59
88	57	0.6	50	0.06	0.05	0.8	53	0	60
93	38	0.4	50	0.03	0.03	0.5	23	0	61

[3] fortified.

Composition per 100 g

No.	Food	Inedible waste %	Energy kcal	Energy kJ	Protein g	Fat g	Carbohydrate (as monosaccharide) g
62	Carrots, old	4	23	98	0.7	0	5.4
63	Cauliflower	30	13	56	1.9	0	1.5
64	Celery	27	8	36	0.9	0	1.3
65	Crisps, potato	0	533	2,224	6.3	35.9	49.3
66	Cucumber	23	9	39	0.6	0	1.8
67	Lentils, dry	0	304	1,293	23.8	1.0	53.2
68	Lettuce	20	9	36	1.0	0	1.2
69	Mushrooms	25	7	31	1.8	0	0
70	Onions	3	23	99	0.9	0	5.2
71	Parsnips	26	49	210	1.7	0	11.3
72	Peas, frozen, raw	0	50	212	5.7	0	7.2
73	Peas, frozen, boiled	0	38	161	5.4	7.7	4.3
74	Peas, canned, processed	35	76	325	6.2	0	13.7
75	Peppers, green	14	12	51	0.9	0	2.2
76	Potatoes, raw	27[6] 14[7]	86	369	2.1	0	20.8
77	Potatoes, boiled	0	79	339	1.4	0	19.7
78	Potato chips, fried	0	253	1,065	3.8	10.9	37.3
79	Potatoes, roast	0	157	662	2.8	4.8	27.3
80	Spinach	25	21	91	2.7	0	2.8
81	Sweet corn, canned	0	76	325	2.9	0.5	16.1
82	Tomatoes, fresh	0	14	60	0.9	0	2.8
83	Turnips	16	17	74	0.8	0	3.8
84	Watercress	23	14	61	2.9	0	0.7
	Fruit						
85	Apples	20	46	196	0.3	0	11.9
86	Apricots, canned (including syrup)	0	106	452	0.5	0	27.7
87	Apricots, dried	0	182	772	4.8	0	43.4
88	Bananas	40	76	326	1.1	0	19.2
89	Blackcurrants	2	28	121	0.9	0	6.6
90	Cherries	13	47	201	0.6	0	11.9
91	Dates, dried	14	248	1,056	2.0	0	63.9
92	Figs, dried	0	213	908	3.6	0	52.9
93	Gooseberries, green	1	17	73	1.1	0	3.4
94	Grapefruit	50	22	95	0.6	0	5.3
95	Lemon juice	64	7	31	0.3	0	1.6
96	Melon	40	23	97	0.8	0	5.2
97	Oranges	25	35	150	0.8	0	8.5

[6] old potatoes [7] new potatoes

Water	Calcium	Iron	Vitamin A (retinol equivalent)	Thia-min	Ribo-flavin	Nicotinic acid equivalent	Vitamin C	Vitamin D	No.
g	mg	mg	μg	mg	mg	mg	mg	μg	
90	48	0.6	2,000	0.06	0.05	0.7	6	0	62
93	21	0.5	5	0.10	0.10	1.1	64	0	63
94	52	0.6	0	0.03	0.03	0.5	7	0	64
3	37	2.1	0	0.19	0.07	6.1	17	0	65
96	23	0.3	0	0.04	0.04	0.3	8	0	66
12	39	7.6	10	0.50	0.20	5.8	0	0	67
96	23	0.9	167	0.07	0.08	0.4	15	0	68
92	3	1.0	0	0.10	0.40	4.6	3	0	69
93	31	0.3	0	0.03	0.05	0.4	10	0	70
83	55	0.6	0	0.10	0.08	1.3	15	0	71
79	33	1.5	50	0.32	0.10	3.0	17	0	72
81	31	1.4	50	0.24	0.07	2.4	13	0	73
72	27	1.5	67	0.10	0.04	1.5	0	0	74
94	9	0.4	33	0.08	0.03	0.9	100	0	75
76	8	0.5	0	0.11	0.04	1.7	8–30[8]	0	76
81	4	0.3	0	0.08	0.03	1.1	5–18[8]	0	77
47	14	0.9	0	0.10	0.04	2.1	6–21[8]		78
64	10	0.7	0	0.10	0.04	1.9	6–21[8]	0	79
91	70	3.2	1,000	0.12	0.20	1.3	60	0	80
73	3	0.6	35	0.05	0.08	0.3	4	0	81
93	13	0.4	100	0.06	0.04	0.8	20[9]	0	82
93	59	0.4	0	0.04	0.05	0.8	25	0	83
91	220	1.6	500	0.10	0.10	1.1	60	0	84
84	4	0.3	5	0.04	0.02	0.1	5	0	85
68	12	0.7	166	0.02	0.01	0.4	2	0	86
15	92	4.1	600	0	0.20	3.8	0	0	87
71	7	0.4	33	0.04	0.07	0.8	10	0	88
77	60	1.3	33	0.03	0.06	0.4	200	0	89
82	16	0.4	20	0.05	0.07	0.4	5	0	90
15	68	1.6	10	0.07	0.04	2.9	0	0	91
17	280	4.2	8	0.10	0.08	2.2	0	0	92
90	28	0.3	30	0.04	0.03	0.5	40	0	93
91	17	0.3	0	0.05	0.02	0.3	40	0	94
91	8	0.1	0	0.02	0.01	0.1	50	0	95
94	16	0.4	175	0.05	0.03	0.5	25	0	96
86	41	0.3	8	0.10	0.03	0.3	50	0	97

[8] vitamin C falls during storage   [9] Feb, 27; May, 14; Aug, 20; Nov, 21 mg per 100 g

Composition per 100 g

No.	Food	Inedible waste %	Energy kcal	kJ	Protein g	Fat g	Carbo-hydrate (as mono-saccharide) g
98	Orange juice, canned, unsweetened	0	33	143	0.4	0	8.5
99	Peaches, fresh	13	37	156	0.6	0	9.1
100	Peaches, canned (including syrup)	0	87	373	0.4	0	22.9
101	Pears, fresh	28	41	175	0.3	0	10.6
102	Pineapple, canned (including syrup)	0	77	328	0.3	0	20.2
103	Plums	8	32	137	0.6	0	7.9
104	Prunes, dried	17	161	686	2.4	0	40.3
105	Raspberries	0	25	105	0.9	0	5.6
106	Rhubarb	33	6	26	0.6	0	1.0
107	Strawberries	3	26	109	0.6	0	6.2
108	Sultanas	0	250	1,066	1.8	0	64.7
	Nuts						
109	Almonds	63	565	2,336	16.9	53.5	4.3
110	Coconut, desiccated	0	604	2,492	5.6	62.0	6.4
111	Peanuts, roasted	0	570	2,364	24.3	49.0	8.6
	Cereals						
112	Barley, pearl, dry	0	360	1,535	7.9	1.7	83.6
113	Biscuits, chocolate	0	524	2,197	5.7	27.6	67.4
114	Biscuits, cream crackers	0	440	1,857	9.5	16.3	68.3
115	Biscuits, plain, semi-sweet	0	457	1,925	6.7	16.6	74.8
116	Biscuits, rich, sweet	0	469	1,966	6.2	23.4	62.2
117	Bread, brown	0	223	948	8.9	2.2	44.7
118	Bread, starch reduced	0	234	996	10.5	1.5	47.6
119	Bread, white	0	233	991	7.8	1.7	49.7
120	Bread, wholemeal	0	216	918	8.8	2.7	41.8
121	Cornflakes	0	368	1,567	8.6	1.6	85.1
122	Custard powder; instant pudding; cornflour	0	354	1,508	0.6	0.7	92.0
123	Crispbread, rye	0	321	1,367	9.4	2.1	70.6
124	Flour, white	0	350	1,493	9.8	1.2	80.1
125	Oatmeal	0	401	1,698	12.4	8.7	72.8
126	Rice	0	361	1,536	6.5	1.0	86.8
127	Spaghetti	0	378	1,612	13.6	1.0	84.0

Water	Calcium	Iron	Vitamin A (retinol equivalent)	Thiamin	Riboflavin	Nicotinic acid equivalent	Vitamin C	Vitamin D	No.
g	mg	mg	μg	mg	mg	mg	mg	μg	
89	9	0.5	8	0.07	0.02	0.3	35	0	98
86	5	0.4	83	0.02	0.05	1.1	8	0	99
74	4	0.4	41	0.01	0.02	0.6	4	0	100
83	8	0.2	2	0.03	0.03	0.3	3	0	101
77	13	0.4	7	0.05	0.02	0.2	12	0	102
85	12	0.3	37	0.05	0.03	0.6	3	0	103
23	38	2.9	160	0.10	0.20	1.9	0	0	104
83	41	1.2	13	0.02	0.03	0.5	25	0	105
94	100	0.4	10	0.01	0.03	0.4	0	0	106
89	22	0.7	5	0.02	0.03	0.5	60	0	107
18	52	1.8	5	0.10	0.08	0.6	0	0	108
5	250	4.2	0	0.24	0.92	4.7	0	0	109
2	22	3.6	0	0.06	0.04	1.8	0	0	110
5	61	2.0	0	0.23	0.10	21.3	0	0	111
11	10	0.7	0	0.12	0.05	2.3	0	0	112
2	110	1.7	0	0.03	0.13	1.4	0	0	113
4	110	1.7	0	0.13	0.08	2.5	0	0	114
3	120	2.1	0	0.13	0.08	2.0	0	0	115
3	87	1.8	0	0.16	0.04	1.7	0	0	116
40	100	2.5	0	0.24	0.06	2.4	0	0	117
36	100	1.3	0	0.18	0.03	2.7	0	0	118
39	100	1.7	0	0.18	0.03	2.2	0	0	119
40	23	2.5	0	0.26	0.06	1.7	0	0	120
3	3	6.7[3]	0	1.80[3]	1.60[3]	21.3[3]	0	2.8[3]	121
		0.6[4]		0[4]	0.03[4]	0.9[4]		0[4]	
12	15	1.4	0	0	0	0.1	0	0	122
6	50	3.7	0	0.28	0.14	1.8	0	0	123
13	150[3]	2.4[3]	0	0.33[3]	0.02	2.8[3]	0	0	124
9	55	4.1	0	0.50	0.10	2.8	0	0	125
12	4	0.5	0	0.08	0.03	1.5	0	0	126
11	23	1.2	0	0.14	0.06	2.8	0	0	127

[3] fortified   [4] unfortified

Composition per 100 g

No.	Food	Inedible waste	Energy		Protein	Fat	Carbo-hydrate (as mono-saccharide)
		%	kcal	kJ	g	g	g
	Beverages						
129	Chocolate, drinking	0	366	1,554	5.5	6.0	77.4
130	Cocoa powder	0	312	1,301	18.5	21.7	11.5
131	Coffee, ground, infusion	0	3	12	0.3	0	0.4
132	Coffee, instant powder	0	100	424	14.6	0	11.0
133	Coca cola	0	39	168	0	0	10.5
134	Tea, dry	0	0	0	0	0	0
135	Squash, fruit, undiluted	0	122	521	0.1	0.1	32.2
	Alcoholic beverages per 100 ml						
136	Beer, keg, bitter	0	31	129	0.3	0	2.3
137	Spirits, 70° proof	0	222	919	0	0	0
138	Wine, red	0	68	284	0.2	0	0.3
	Puddings and cakes etc.						
139	Apple pie	0	281	1,179	3.2	14.4	40.4
140	Bread and butter pudding	0	154	649	5.3	7.1	18.5
141	Buns, currant	0	328	1,385	7.8	8.5	58.6
142	Custard	0	118	496	3.8	4.4	16.8
143	Fruit cake, rich	0	332	1,403	3.7	11.0	58.3
144	Jam tarts	0	384	1,616	3.5	14.9	62.8
145	Plain cake, Madeira	0	393	1,652	5.4	16.9	58.4
146	Rice pudding	0	131	552	4.1	4.2	20.2
147	Soup, tomato, canned	0	55	230	0.8	3.3	5.9
148	Trifle	0	160	674	3.5	6.1	24.3
149	Marmite	0	172	730	39.7	0.7	1.8
150	Ice-cream, vanilla	0	166	698	3.5	7.4	22.8

Water	Calcium	Iron	Vitamin A (retinol equivalent)	Thia-min	Ribo-flavin	Nicotinic acid equivalent	Vitamin C	Vitamin D	No.
g	mg	mg	μg	mg	mg	mg	mg	μg	
2	33	2.4	2	0.06	0.04	2.1	0	0	129
3	130	10.5	7	0.16	0.06	7.3	0	0	130
—	3	0	0	0	0.20	10.0	0	0	131
3	160	4.4	0	0	0.11	25.1	0	0	132
90	4	0	0	0	0	0	0	0	133
—	0	0	0	0	0.90[10]	6.0[10]	0	0	134
63	16	0.2	0	0	0.01	0	1	0	135
—	8	0	0	0	0.03	0.5	0	0	136
—	0	0	0	0	0	0	0	0	137
—	7	0.9	0	0.01	0.02	0.1	0	0	138
42	42	0.8	2	0.08	0.02	0.9	2	0	139
67	112	0.7	79	0.06	0.22	1.5	1.5	0.30	140
25	88	1.6	24	0.15	0.10	2.0	0	0.27	141
75	140	0.1	43	0.05	0.21	1.0	0	0.03	142
21	75	1.8	121	0.08	0.08	1.2	0	1.14	143
19	62	1.6	0	0.08	0.01	1.1	4	0	144
20	42	1.1	82	0.06	0.11	1.4	0	1.20	145
72	130	0.1	33	0.04	0.14	1.1	1	0.02	146
84	17	0.4	35	0.03	0.02	0.2	0	0	147
65	82	0.7	60	0.05	0.14	1.0	1	0.17	148
25	95	3.7	0	3.10	11.00	67.0	0	0	149
65	130	0.3	7	0.04	0.17	1.0	1	0	150

[10] 90 to 100 per cent is extracted into an infusion

Table 2. **Composition per oz (raw edible weight except where stated)**

No.	Food	Inedible waste %	Energy kcal	Energy kJ	Protein g	Fat g	Cargo-hydrate (as mono-saccharide) g
	Milk						
1	Cream, double	0	127	522	0.4	13.7	0.6
2	Cream, single	0	55	229	0.7	5.5	0.9
3	Milk, liquid, whole	0	18	77	0.9	1.1	1.3
4	Milk, condensed, whole, sweetened	0	91	386	2.4	2.6	15.7
5	Milk, whole, evaporated	0	45	187	2.4	2.6	3.2
6	Milk, UHT	0	18	78	0.9	1.1	1.3
7	Milk, dried, skimmed	0	101	429	10.3	0.4	15.0
8	Yogurt, low-fat, natural	0	15	61	1.4	0.3	1.8
9	Yogurt, low-fat, fruit	0	27	115	1.4	0.3	5.1
	Cheese						
10	Cheese, Cheddar	0	115	477	7.4	9.5	0
11	Cheese, cottage	0	27	114	3.8	1.1	0.4
	Meat						
12	Bacon, rashers, raw	11	120	494	4.1	11.5	0
13	Bacon, rashers, cooked	0	127	525	6.9	11.0	0
14	Beef, average, raw	17	75	314	4.9	6.2	0
15	Beef, corned	0	62	255	7.6	3.4	0
16	Beef, stewing steak, raw	3	48	202	5.6	2.9	0
17	Beef, stewing steak, cooked	0	63	264	8.8	3.1	0
18	Black pudding	0	87	361	3.7	6.2	4.3
19	Chicken, raw	33	65	270	5.0	5.0	0
20	Chicken, roast, light meat	0	40	170	7.5	1.1	0
21	Ham, cooked	0	77	319	7.0	5.4	0
22	Kidney, average	12	26	108	4.6	0.8	0
23	Lamb, average, raw	17	95	395	4.5	8.6	0
24	Lamb, roast	25	83	344	6.5	6.3	0
25	Liver, average, raw	0	46	193	5.9	2.3	0.6
26	Liver, fried	0	69	288	7.1	3.8	1.6
27	Luncheon meat	0	89	368	3.6	7.6	1.6
28	Pork, average, raw	26	92	381	4.5	8.2	0
29	Pork chop, grilled	22	94	393	8.1	6.9	0
30	Sausage, pork	0	104	431	3.0	9.1	2.7
31	Sausage, beef	0	84	350	2.7	6.8	3.3
32	Steak and kidney pie, cooked	0	81	339	4.3	5.2	4.6
33	Tripe, dressed	0	17	72	2.7	0.7	0

Calcium mg	Iron mg	Vitamin A (retinol equivalent) μg	Thiamin mg	Ribo-flavin mg	Nicotinic acid equivalent mg	Vitamin C mg	Vitamin D μg	No.
14	0.1	142	0.01	0.02	0.1	0	0.08	1
22	0.1	44	0.01	0.03	0.2	0	0.04	2
34	0	13[1] 9[2]	0.01	0.05	0.3	0	0.03 [1] 0.01[2]	3
79	0.1	35	0.02	0.14	0.6	1	0.02	4
79	0.1	31	0.02	0.14	0.6	0	0.82 [3]	5
34	0	11	0.01	0.05	0.2	0	0.01	6
337	0.1	0	0.12	0.45	2.8	2	0	7
51	0	3	0.01	0.07	0.3	0	0	8
45	0.1	6	0.01	0.07	0.3	1	0	9
227	0.1	117	0.01	0.14	1.8	0	0.07	10
17	0	12	0	0.05	0.9	0	0.01	11
3	0.3	0	0.10	0.04	1.7	0	0	12
3	0.4	0	0.11	0.05	2.6	0	0	13
2	0.5	0	0.01	0.05	2.1	0	0	14
4	0.8	0	0	0.07	2.5	0	0	15
2	0.6	0	0.02	0.06	2.4	0	0	16
4	0.8	0	0.01	0.09	2.9	0	0	17
10	6.0	0	0.03	0.02	1:1	0	0	18
3	0.2	0	0.02	0.04	2.6	0	0	19
3	0.1	0	0.02	0.04	4.3	0	0	20
3	0.4	0	0.13	0.04	2.3	0	0	21
2	1.7	34	0.11	0.54	3.0	3	0	22
2	0.4	0	0.02	0.05	2.1	0	0	23
2	0.6	0	0.02	0.07	2.6	0	0	24
2	3.2	4,160	0.07	0.88	5.1	4	0.21	25
4	2.5	5,390	0.07	1.20	5.8	3	0.11	26
4	0.3	0	0.02	0.03	1.3	0	0	27
2	0.2	0	0.17	0.05	2.0	0	0	28
3	0.3	0	0.19	0.06	3.1	0	0	29
12	0.3	0	0.01	0.03	1.6	0	0	30
14	0.4	0	0.01	0.04	2.0	0	0	31
10	0.8	36	0.04	0.15	1.9	1	0.16	32
21	0.2	0	0	0	0.6	0	0	33

[1] Summer value [2] Winter value [3] fortified

Composition per oz

No.	Food	Inedible waste %	Energy kcal	kJ	Protein g	Fat g	Carbo-hydrate (as mono-saccharide) g
	Fish						
34	White fish, filleted	5	21	91	4.9	0.2	0
35	Cod, fried in batter	0	56	236	5.6	2.9	2.1
36	Fish fingers	0	51	212	3.6	2.1	4.6
37	Herring	37	66	274	4.8	5.2 [5]	0
38	Kipper fillets	2	52	217	5.6	3.3 [5]	0
39	Salmon, canned	6	44	184	5.8	2.3	0
40	Sardines, canned in oil, fish only	7	62	258	6.7	3.9	0
	Eggs						
41	Eggs, fresh	12	42	174	3.5	3.1	0
	Fats						
42	Butter	0	210	862	0.1	23.2	0
43	Lard; cooking fat; dripping	0	253	1,040	0	28.1	0
44	Low-fat spread	0	104	427	0	11.5	0
45	Margarine, average	0	207	851	0	23.0	0
46	Oils, cooking and salad	0	255	1,047	0	28.3	0
	Preserves etc						
47	Chocolate, milk	0	150	628	2.4	8.6	16.8
48	Honey	0	82	349	0.1	0	21.7
49	Jam	0	74	315	0.1	0	19.6
50	Marmalade	0	74	315	0	0	19.7
51	Sugar, white	0	112	477	0	0	29.8
52	Syrup	0	84	360	0.1	0	22.4
	Vegetables						
53	Beans, canned in tomato sauce	0	18	76	1.4	0.1	2.9
54	Beans, broad	75	19	81	2.0	0.1	2.7
55	Beans, haricot, dry	0	77	326	6.1	0.4	12.9
56	Beans, runner	14	7	29	0.6	0	1.1
57	Beetroot, boiled	20	12	53	0.5	0	2.8
58	Brussels sprouts, raw	25	7	32	1.1	0	0.8
59	Brussels sprouts, boiled	0	5	22	0.8	0	0.5
60	Cabbage, green, raw	30	6	26	0.8	0	0.8
61	Cabbage, green, boiled	0	5	20	0.5	0	0.7

[5] Fat content varies throughout the year between 10 and 25 per cent.

Calcium	Iron	Vitamin A (retinol equivalent)	Thiamin	Ribo-flavin	Nicotinic acid equivalent	Vitamin C	Vitamin D	No.
mg	mg	μg	mg	mg	mg	mg	μg	
5	0.1	0	0.02	0.02	1.4	0	0	34
23	0.1	0	0.01	0.03	1.9	0	0	35
12	0.2	0	0.03	0.02	0.9	0	0	36
9	0.2	13	0	0.05	2.0	0	6.40	37
17	0.3	13	0.01	0.09	2.0	0	6.38	38
26	0.4	26	0.01	0.05	3.1	0	3.54	39
156	0.8	0	0.01	0.10	3.6	0	2.12	40
15	0.6	40	0.02	0.13	1.1	0	0.50	41
4	0	279	0	0	0	0	0.22	42
0	0	0	0	0	0	0	0	43
0	0	255 [3]	0	0	0	0	2.25 [3]	44
1	0.1	255 [3]	0	0	0	0	2.25 [3]	45
0	0	0	0	0	0	0	0	46
62	0.4	2	0.03	0.06	0.4	0	0	47
1	0.1	0	0	0.01	0.1	0	0	48
5	0.3	1	0	0	0	3	0	49
10	0.2	2	0	0	0	3	0	50
1	0	0	0	0	0	0	0	51
7	0.4	0	0	0	0	0	0	52
13	0.4	14	0.02	0.01	0.4	0	0	53
9	0.3	6	0.08	0.01	1.4	9	0	54
51	1.9	0	0.13	0.04	1.7	0	0	55
8	0.2	14	0.01	0.03	0.4	6	0	56
9	0.2	0	0	0.01	0.1	1	0	57
9	0.2	19	0.03	0.04	0.4	25	0	58
7	0.2	19	0.02	0.03	0.3	10	0	59
16	0.2	14	0.02	0.01	0.2	15	0	60
11	0.1	14	0.01	0.01	0.1	6	0	61

[3] fortified

Composition per oz

No.	Food	Inedible waste %	Energy kcal	kJ	Protein g	Fat g	Carbo-hydrate (as mono-saccharide) g
62	Carrots, old	4	6	27	0.2	0	1.5
63	Cauliflower	30	4	15	0.5	0	0.4
64	Celery	27	3	12	0.3	0	0.4
65	Crisps, potato	0	152	631	1.8	10.2	14.0
66	Cucumber	23	2	8	0.1	0	0.4
67	Lentils, dry	0	86	366	6.8	0.3	15.1
68	Lettuce	20	3	10	0.3	0	0.3
69	Mushrooms	25	2	9	0.5	0	0
70	Onions	3	7	28	0.3	0	1.5
71	Parsnips	26	14	60	0.5	0	3.2
72	Peas, frozen, raw	0	14	60	1.6	0	2.0
73	Peas, frozen, boiled	0	11	46	1.5	0	1.2
74	Peas, canned, processed	35	22	93	1.8	0	3.9
75	Peppers, green	14	3	14	0.3	0	0.6
76	Potatoes, raw	27[6] 14[7]	24	105	0.6	0	5.9
77	Potatoes, boiled	0	22	96	0.4	0	5.6
78	Potato chips, fried	0	72	302	1.1	3.1	10.6
79	Potatoes, roast	0	44	188	0.8	1.4	7.7
80	Spinach	25	6	26	0.8	0	0.8
81	Sweet corn, canned	0	22	92	0.8	0.1	4.6
82	Tomatoes, fresh	0	4	17	0.2	0	0.8
83	Turnips	16	5	21	0.2	0	1.1
84	Watercress	23	4	17	0.8	0	0.2
	Fruit						
85	Apples	20	13	56	0.1	0	3.4
86	Apricots, canned (including syrup)	0	30	128	0.1	0	7.9
87	Apricots, dried	0	52	221	1.4	0	12.3
88	Bananas	40	22	93	0.3	0	5.5
89	Blackcurrants	2	8	36	0.3	0	1.9
90	Cherries	13	13	57	0.2	0	3.4
91	Dates, dried	14	70	300	0.6	0	18.1
92	Figs, dried	0	60	257	1.0	0	15.0
93	Gooseberries, green	1	5	21	0.3	0	1.0
94	Grapefruit	50	6	27	0.2	0	1.5
95	Lemon juice	64	2	10	0.1	0	0.5
96	Melon	40	6	27	0.2	0	1.5
97	Oranges	25	10	42	0.2	0	2.4

[6] old potatoes   [7] new potatoes

Calcium mg	Iron mg	Vitamin A (retinol equivalent) μg	Thiamin mg	Ribo-flavin mg	Nicotinic acid equivalent mg	Vitamin C mg	Vitamin D μg	No.
14	0.2	567	0.02	0.01	0.2	2	0	62
6	0.1	1	0.03	0.03	0.3	18	0	63
15	0.2	0	0.01	0.01	0.1	2	0	64
10	0.6	0	0.05	0.02	1.7	5	0	65
5	0.1	0	0.01	0.01	0.1	2	0	66
11	2.2	3	0.14	0.06	1.6	0	0	67
6	0.3	47	0.02	0.02	0.1	4	0	68
1	0.3	0	0.03	0.11	1.3	1	0	69
9	0.1	0	0.01	0.01	0.1	3	0	70
16	0.2	0	0.03	0.02	0.4	4	0	71
9	0.4	14	0.09	0.03	0.8	5	0	72
9	0.4	14	0.07	0.02	0.7	4	0	73
8	0.4	19	0.03	0.01	0.4	0	0	74
2	0.1	9	0	0.01	0.2	28	0	75
2	0.1	0	0.03	0.01	0.5	2−9[8]	0	76
1	0.1	0	0.02	0.01	0.3	1−5[8]	0	77
4	0.2	0	0.03	0.01	0.6	2−6[8]	0	78
3	0.2	0	0.03	0.01	0.5	2−6[8]	0	79
20	0.9	284	0.03	0.06	0.4	17	0	80
1	0.2	10	0.01	0.02	0.1	1	0	81
4	0.1	28	0.02	0.01	0.2	6	0	82
17	0.1	0	0.01	0.01	0.2	7	0	83
62	0.5	142	0.03	0.03	0.3	17	0	84
1	0.1	1	0.01	0.01	0	1	0	85
3	0.2	47	0.01	0	0.1	1	0	86
26	1.2	170	0	0.06	1.1	0	0	87
2	0.1	9	0.01	0.02	0.2	3	0	88
17	0.4	9	0.01	0.02	0.1	57	0	89
4	0.1	6	0.01	0.02	0.1	1	0	90
19	0.5	3	0.02	0.01	0.8	0	0	91
79	1.2	2	0.03	0.02	0.6	0	0	92
8	0.1	9	0.01	0.01	0.1	11	0	93
5	0.1	0	0.01	0.01	0.1	11	0	94
2	0	0	0.01	0	0	14	0	95
5	0.1	50	0.01	0.01	0.1	7	0	96
12	0.1	2	0.03	0.01	0.1	14	0	97

[8] vitamin C falls during storage

Composition per oz

No.	Food	Inedible waste %	Energy kcal	kJ	Protein g	Fat g	Carbo-hydrate (as mono-saccharide) g
98	Orange juice, canned, unsweetened	0	9	41	0.1	0	2.4
99	Peaches, fresh	13	10	45	0.2	0	2.6
100	Peaches, canned (including syrup)	0	25	106	0.1	0	6.5
101	Pears, fresh	28	12	50	0.1	0	3.0
102	Pineapple, canned (including syrup)	0	22	93	0.1	0	5.7
103	Plums	8	9	39	0.2	0	2.2
104	Prunes, dried	17	46	194	0.7	0	11.4
105	Raspberries	0	7	31	0.3	0	1.6
106	Rhubarb	33	2	8	0.2	0	0.3
107	Strawberries	3	8	32	0.2	0	1.8
108	Sultanas	0	71	302	0.5	0	18.3
	Nuts						
109	Almonds	63	160	662	4.8	15.2	1.2
110	Coconut, desiccated	0	171	706	1.6	17.6	1.8
111	Peanuts, roasted	0	162	670	6.9	13.9	2.4
	Cereals						
112	Barley, pearl, dry	0	102	435	2.2	0.5	23.7
113	Biscuits, chocolate	0	148	623	1.6	7.8	19.1
114	Biscuits, cream crackers	0	125	526	2.7	4.6	19.4
115	Biscuits, plain, semi-sweet	0	130	546	1.9	4.7	21.2
116	Biscuits, rich, sweet	0	133	557	1.8	6.6	17.6
117	Bread, brown	0	63	269	2.5	0.6	12.7
118	Bread, starch reduced	0	66	282	3.0	0.4	13.5
119	Bread, white	0	66	281	2.2	0.5	14.1
120	Bread, wholemeal	0	61	260	2.5	0.8	11.8
121	Cornflakes	0	104	444	2.4	0.4	24.1
122	Custard powder; instant pudding; cornflour	0	100	428	0.2	0.2	26.1
123	Crispbread, rye	0	91	388	2.7	0.6	20.0
124	Flour, white	0	99	423	2.8	0.3	22.7
125	Oatmeal	0	114	481	3.5	2.5	20.6
126	Rice	0	102	435	1.8	0.3	24.6
127	Spaghetti	0	107	457	3.8	0.3	23.8

Calcium mg	Iron mg	Vitamin A (retinol equivalent) μg	Thiamin mg	Ribo-flavin mg	Nicotinic acid equivalent mg	Vitamin C mg	Vitamin D μg	No.
3	0.1	2	0.02	0.01	0.1	10	0	98
1	0.1	24	0.01	0.01	0.3	2	0	99
1	0.1	12	0	0.01	0.2	1	0	100
2	0.1	1	0.01	0.01	0.1	1	0	101
4	0.1	2	0.01	0.01	0.1	3	0	102
3	0.1	10	0.01	0.01	0.2	1	0	103
11	0.8	45	0.03	0.06	0.5	0	0	104
12	0.3	4	0.01	0.01	7	0	0	105
28	0.1	3	0	0.01	0.1	3	0	106
6	0.2	1	0.01	0.01	0.1	17	0	107
15	0.5	1	0.03	0.02	0.2	0	0	108
71	1.2	0	0.07	0.26	1.3	0	0	109
6	1.0	0	0.02	0.01	0.5	0	0	110
17	0.6	0	0.07	0.03	6.0	0	0	111
3	0.2	0	0.03	0.01	0.6	0	0	112
31	0.5	0	0.01	0.04	0.4	0	0	113
31	0.5	0	0.04	0.02	0.7	0	0	114
34	0.6	0	0.04	0.02	0.6	0	0	115
25	0.5	0	0.04	0.01	0.5	0	0	116
28	0.7	0	0.07	0.02	0.7	0	0	117
28	0.4	0	0.05	0.01	0.8	0	0	118
28	0.5	0	0.05	0.01	0.6	0	0	119
6	0.7	0	0.07	0.02	0.5	0	0	120
1	1.90[3]	0	0.50[3]	0.40[3]	6.0[3]	0	0.8[3]	121
	0.2[4]		0[4]	0[4]	0.3[4]		0[4]	
4	0.4	0	0	0	0	0	0	122
14	1.0	0	0.08	0.04	0.5	0	0	123
42[3]	0.7[3]	0	0.09[3]	0.01	0.8[3]	0	0	124
16	1.2	0	0.14	0.03	0.8	0	0	125
1	0.1	0	0.02	0.01	0.4	0	0	126
6	0.3	0	0.04	0.02	0.8	0	0	127

[3] fortified   [4] unfortified

117

Composition per oz

No.	Food	Inedible waste	Energy		Protein	Fat	Carbohydrate (as monosaccharide)
		%	kcal	kJ	g	g	g
	Beverages						
129	Chocolate, drinking	0	104	441	1.6	1.7	21.9
130	Cocoa powder	0	88	369	5.2	6.2	3.3
131	Coffee, ground, infusion	0	1	3	0.1	0	0.1
132	Coffee, instant powder	0	28	120	4.1	0	3.1
133	Coca cola	0	11	48	0	0	3.0
134	Tea, dry	0	0	0	0	0	0
135	Squash, fruit, undiluted	0	34	146	0	0	9.1
	Alcoholic beverages per fl oz						
136	Beer, keg bitter	0	9	37	0.1	0	0.6
137	Spirits, 70° proof	0	63	261	0	0	0
138	Wine, red	0	19	80	0.1	0	0.1
	Puddings and cakes etc.						
139	Apple pie	0	80	336	0.9	4.1	11.5
140	Bread and butter pudding	0	44	184	1.5	2.0	5.2
141	Buns, currant	0	93	392	2.2	2.4	16.6
142	Custard	0	33	141	1.1	1.2	4.8
143	Fruit cake, rich	0	94	398	1.0	3.1	16.5
144	Jam tarts	0	109	458	1.0	4.2	17.8
145	Plain cake, Madeira	0	111	468	1.5	4.8	16.6
146	Rice pudding	0	37	156	1.2	1.2	5.8
147	Soup, tomato, canned	0	16	65	0.2	0.9	1.7
148	Trifle	0	45	191	1.0	1.7	6.9
149	Marmite	0	49	207	11.2	0.2	0.5
150	Ice-cream, vanilla	0	47	198	1.0	2.1	6.5

Calcium mg	Iron mg	Vitamin A (retinol equivalent) μg	Thiamin mg	Ribo-flavin mg	Nicotinic acid equivalent mg	Vitamin C mg	Vitamin D μg	No.
9	0.7	0.6	0.02	0.01	0.6	0	0	129
37	3.0	2	0.04	0.02	2.1	0	0	130
1	0	0	0	0.06	2.8	0	0	131
45	1.2	0	0	0.03	7.1	0	0	132
1	0	0	0	0	0	0	0	133
0	0	0	0	0.30[10]	1.7[10]	0	0	134
5	0.1	0	0	0	0	0	0	135
2	0	0	0	0.01	0.1	0	0	136
0	0	0	0	0	0	0	0	137
2	0.2	0	0	0.10	0	0	0	138
12	0.2	1	0.02	0.01	0.3	1	0	139
32	0.2	23	0.02	0.06	0.4	0	0.08	140
25	0.5	7	0.04	0.03	0.6	0	0.08	141
40	0	12	0.01	0.06	0.3	0	0.01	142
21	0.5	34	0.02	0.02	0.3	0	0.32	143
18	0.4	0	0.02	0	0.3	1	0	144
12	0.3	23	0.01	0.03	0.4	0	0.34	145
37	0	9	0.01	0.04	0.3	0	0	146
5	0.1	10	0.01	0.01	0.1	0	0	147
23	0.2	17	0.01	0.04	0.3	1	0.05	148
27	1.0	0	0.90	3.10	19.4	0	0	149
37	0.1	2	0.01	0.05	0.3	0	0	150

[10] 90 to 100 per cent extracted into an infusion

3 The use of food tables for calculations on the nutritional value of foods

A great deal of useful information can be worked out from the food composition tables in Appendix 2. Examples of various types of calculation are given below:

1. NUTRIENT CONTENT

(a) *Simple nutrient content*
To calculate the protein content of 4 oz *fish fingers*
Item 36, Table 2: Fish fingers contain 3.6 g protein per oz
∴ 4 oz raw fish fingers contain 3.6 x 4
$= 14.4$ g protein

(b) *Nutrient content allowing for wastage (inedible matter)*
To calculate the vitamin A content of 200 g *fresh whole peaches*
Item 99, Table 1: Peaches contain 83 μg vitamin A per 100 g (raw, edible portion) and 13 per cent waste.

$$200 \text{ g whole peaches contain } (\frac{100-13}{100}) \times 200 \text{ g edible matter}$$

$$= 174 \text{ g edible matter}$$

$$\text{Therefore 200 g whole peaches contain } \frac{174}{100} \times 83$$

$$= 144 \text{ μg vitamin A}$$

2. PORTION SIZES

(a) *100 Kilocalorie portions*
e.g., *Black pudding*
Item 18, Table 1: Black pudding has an energy value of 305 kcal per 100 g

$$∴ 100 \text{ kcal are contained in } \frac{100}{305} \times 100$$

$$= 33 \text{ g (or just over 1 oz) black pudding}$$

Lettuce

Item 68, Table 1: Lettuce has an energy value of 9 kcal per 100 g

∴ 100 kcal are contained in $\dfrac{100}{9}$ x 100

= 1,111 g (nearly $2\frac{1}{2}$ lb) lettuce

(b) *400 Kilojoule portions* (The size of a 400 kJ portion will be slightly smaller than a 100 kcal portion, while a 500 kJ portion will be larger)

e.g., *Butter*

Item 42, Table 1: Butter has an energy value of 3,041 kJ per 100 g

∴ 400 kJ are contained in $\dfrac{400}{3,041}$ x 100

= 13 g (less than $\frac{1}{2}$ oz) butter

Boiled potatoes

Item 77, Table 1: Boiled potatoes have an energy value of 339 kJ per 100 g

∴ 400 kJ are contained in $\dfrac{400}{339}$ x 100

= 118 g (about 4 oz) boiled potatoes

(c) *Portion sizes in relation to recommended intakes*

To calculate the *weight of beef supplying one-third of the recommended daily intake* (RDI) *of nicotinic acid equivalents for a woman.*

One-third of the RDI = 5 mg (page 54).

Item 14, Table 1 gives 7.3 mg nicotinic acid equivalent per 100 g edible portion

∴ 5 mg are contained in $\dfrac{5}{7.3}$ x 100

= 68 g (about $2\frac{1}{2}$ oz) edible beef

Also, since on average beef has 17 per cent inedible matter, 100 g beef as purchased contain 100–17

= 83 g edible beef

∴ 62 g edible beef are contained in $\dfrac{68}{83}$ x 100

= 82 g (nearly 3 oz) beef, weighed with bone

3. COST OF NUTRIENTS

(a) *Nutrients bought per penny*

To calculate the nutrients obtained per penny from a small (14 oz) loaf of *white bread* costing 16p

1p buys $\dfrac{14}{16}$

= 0.9 oz bread

Item 119 in Table 2 (per oz) is white bread.
Therefore multiply the values for each nutrient by 0.9
$\quad$=2.0 g protein
$\quad$=0.4 g fat
$\quad$=12.7 g carbohydrate
$\quad$=25 mg calcium
$\quad$=0.4 mg iron etc.

(b) *Where foods are purchased without inedible matter*
To calculate the cost of 10 g protein from *Cheddar cheese* at 65p per lb
Item 10, Table 2: Cheddar cheese contains 7.4 g protein per oz

Therefore 10 g protein are contained in $\dfrac{10}{7.4}$ x 1

$$=1.35 \text{ oz cheese}$$

Cost of 1.35 oz cheese $=1.35 \times \dfrac{65}{16}$

$$=5.5\text{p}$$

(c) *Where foods are purchased with inedible matter*
To calculate the cost of 15 mg vitamin C from *green peppers* at 40 p per lb
Item 75, Table 2: Green peppers contain 28 mg vitamin C per oz of edible portion, and 14 per cent waste

Therefore 15 mg vitamin C are contained in $\dfrac{15}{28}$ x 1

$$=0.54 \text{ oz peppers (edible portion)}$$

Because of the wastage of seeds and stalk,

1oz of peppers as purchased $=\dfrac{\cdot100-14}{100}$ oz edible portion

or 1 oz peppers, edible portion $=\dfrac{100}{100-14}$ oz as purchased

∴ 0.54 oz (edible portion) $=0.63$ oz as purchased

Cost of 0.63 oz $=0.63 \times \dfrac{40}{16}$

$$=1.6\text{p}$$

4 Average weights and measures of commonly used foods

Milk	for { 1 cup of tea	1 oz
	{ 1 glass	7 oz
Cheese	1″ cube	$\frac{3}{4}$ oz
Steak	average	6–8 oz
Bacon	1 large rasher	1 oz
Sausage	1 large sausage	2 oz
Meat pie	1 individual pie	4 oz
Eggs	1 egg	2 oz or 50 g
Butter or margarine	for 1 slice bread	$\frac{1}{8}$–$\frac{1}{4}$ oz
Lettuce	2 large leaves	$\frac{1}{2}$ oz
Potatoes, boiled	2 medium	4 oz
mashed	1 scoop	2 oz
Tomato	2 medium size	3 oz
Orange	1 medium (with peel)	4 oz
Apple	1 medium	3 oz
Bread	1 thick slice from small loaf	1 oz
	1 thick slice from large loaf	2 oz
Flour	1 tablespoon, rounded	1 oz
Porridge oats	1 tea cup	3 oz
Breakfast cereal	1 helping	$\frac{3}{4}$–1 oz
Biscuits, dry	three	1 oz
plain sweet	one	$\frac{1}{3}$ oz
Coffee, instant	per cup	$\frac{1}{10}$ oz or 2 g
Tea	per cup	$\frac{1}{6}$ oz
Beer	$\frac{1}{2}$ pint	10 fl oz or 285 ml
Wine	1 wineglass	$2\frac{1}{2}$ fl oz or 70 ml

5 Food additives

In addition to the expected ingredients of made-up foods there are other substances which may be added in small amounts to perform a special function in the food. These are called *food additives*. They fall into two broad categories: those which are added to prevent food spoilage and those which are added to enhance the texture, flavour or appearance of food.

Preservatives and antioxidants
It is very important that every effort is made to prevent sound food being wasted. Some forms of food spoilage, such as attacks on stored food by vermin, are easily recognized. Other forms of spoilage develop within the food itself and give rise to off-flavours long before the visual appearance of the food is noticeably affected; these may arise either by the action of micro-organisms (i.e., moulds and bacteria) or by chemical action. While some micro-organisms merely make the food unpalatable, others such as *Clostridium botulinum* produce highly poisonous toxins and present a considerable hazard to health. Preservatives such as sulphur dioxide and sodium nitrite are added to some foods to inhibit the growth of micro-organisms. The most common form of chemical spoilage is rancidity. Rancidity resulting from the oxidation of fat can be retarded by the addition of antioxidants. Some antioxidants are natural compounds but in order to protect fat in foods which are baked, e.g. biscuits, heat-stable synthetic antioxidants are required.

Other additives
The texture of food often depends on the ability of added emulsifiers to form a uniform dispersion of fat and water e.g., in margarine. Similarly, stabilizers are added to prevent uniform dispersions separating out e.g., in the setting of instant desserts.

The colour and flavour of foods are closely linked: consumers expect a food to have a colour which matches the flavour. Therefore, if the natural colour is lost or changed during processing, colouring matter may be added to restore the food to the expected colour.

The law strictly controls the main classes of additives which may be used in food. (See also Appendix 6).

6 Legislation governing the composition and labelling of food

The major piece of legislation in this field is the *Food and Drugs Act 1955*. Legislation is made jointly by the Minister of Agriculture and the Secretary of State for Social Services. This applies only in England and Wales, but there is similar legislation in Scotland and Northern Ireland.

The most important provisions of the Act are: (a) to make it an offence to sell to the prejudice of the purchaser food which is not of the nature, substance or quality demanded, (b) to prohibit the use of a 'label or advertisement which falsely describes a food or misleads as to its nature, substance or quality, (c) to prohibit the addition to or abstraction of any substance from food so as to render the food injurious to health, and (d) make it an offence to sell unsound food. These general provisions are backed up by many regulations which lay down detailed requirements as to the labelling of all foods, the composition of the major foods (as below) in our diet, and the type and level of additives and contaminants permitted in food.

Ministers are advised on the need for and type of regulations by the Food Standards Committee (on compositional and labelling matters) and by the Food Additives and Contaminants Committee. Both Committees consult all interested parties, including consumers, enforcement officers and the food industries before coming to any decisions. Before making regulations, Ministers are again required to consult all those interested.

The Labelling of Food Regulations 1970 (As Amended) require most prepacked foods to bear a common or usual name or an appropriate designation of the food, a list of ingredients in descending order by weight, and the name and address of the packer or labeller (or somebody resident in the United Kingdom who is responsible for the food). These regulations also control claims on the label or in advertising that, for example, the food will provide energy or protein, is an aid to slimming, or will be useful to diabetics. Vitamin and mineral claims may only be made for the following nutrients: vitamin A, thiamin, riboflavin, nicotinic acid, vitamin C, vitamin D, iron, calcium and iodine.

The compositional regulations lay down standards for certain foods; for example, minimum meat contents are linked to certain permitted names in the many meat products regulations. A pork sausage, for instance, under the *Sausage and Other Meat Product Regulations 1967 (As Amended)* must contain 65 per cent meat but a beef sausage only 50 per cent.

Detailed requirements are laid down for the composition of bread by the *Bread and Flour Regulations 1963 (As Amended)*. The use of colouring matter is restricted, the permitted bleaching and improving agents listed, minimum nutrient levels for flour are prescribed, and the amount of chalk which must be added to all flour except self-raising, wholemeal and wheat malt flour laid down (see also page 75).

The *Margarine Regulations 1967* require, amongst other things, that all margarine for retail sale must be fortified with vitamins A and D and that this must be declared on the label (see also page 67).

The additive regulations lay down lists of permitted additives and standards of purity. The safety of additives, and the need for their use, is given full and detailed consideration before they are permitted to be used in food. Existing regulations control, for example, preservatives, colouring matters, antioxidants, and emulsifiers and stabilizers. Food contaminants such as heavy metals are also strictly controlled by legislation.

The full Regulations, which are obtainable from Her Majesty's Stationery Office, should be consulted for further information.

7 Books for further reading

W Matthews and D Wells. *Second Book of Food and Nutrition.* 3rd ed. London: Home Economics and Flour Advisory Bureau, 1976.
(ISBN 0 90 176223 7)

M Pyke, *Success in Nutrition.* London: John Murray, 1975.
(ISBN 0 71 953186 1)

Sir S Davidson, R Passmore, J F Brock and A S Truswell. *Human Nutrition and Dietetics.* 6th revised ed. Edinburgh: Churchill Livingstone, 1975.
Paper (ISBN 0 44 301310 1)
Cloth (ISBN 0 44 301246 6)

H M Sinclair and D F Hollingsworth (eds). *Hutchison's Food and the Principles of Nutrition.* 12th ed. London: Edward Arnold, 1969.
(ISBN 0 71 314139 5)

A E Bender. *Dictionary of Nutrition and Food Technology.* 4th ed. London: Newnes – Butterworth, 1975.
(ISBN 0 40 800143 7)

Ministry of Agriculture, Fisheries and Food. *Household Food Consumption and Expenditure 1976: Annual Report of the National Food Survey Committee.* London: HMSO, 1977.
(ISBN 0 11 241052 9)

J C Drummond and A Wilbraham. *The Englishman's Food: A History of Five Centuries of English Diet.* Revised and with a new chapter by D Hollingsworth. London: Johnathan Cape, 1958.
(ISBN 0 22 460168 7)

M E Lowenberg, E N Todhunter, E D Wilson, J R Savage and J L Lubwaski. *Food and Man.* 2nd ed. Chichester: Wiley, 1974.
(ISBN 0 47 154961 4)

D Hollingsworth and M Russell (eds). *Nutritional Problems in a Changing World.* London: Applied Science, 1973.
(ISBN 0 85 334581 3)

G Borgstrom. *World Food Resources.* London: Intertext Books, 1973.
(ISBN 0 70 020229 3)

M Gunther. *Infant Feeding.* Harmondsworth: Penguin, 1973.
(ISBN 0 14 046197 3)

Department of Health and Social Security. *Present-Day Practice in Infant Feeding*. Report on Health and Social Subjects 9. London: HMSO, 1974.

(ISBN 0 11 320581 3)

B Nilson. *Cooking for Special Diets*. Harmondsworth: Penguin, 1972.

(ISBN 0 14 046095 0)

Department of Health and Social Security. *Diet and Coronary Heart Disease*. Report on Health and Social Subjects 7. London: HMSO, 1974.

(ISBN 0 11 320507 4)

Swedish Nutrition Foundation. *Nutrition in Old Age*. Symposia of the Swedish Nutrition Foundation X. Uppsala: The Foundation, 1972.

J V G A Durnin and R Passmore. *Energy, Work and Leisure*. London: Heinemann Educational, 1967.

(ISBN 0 43 562270 6)

World Health Organization. *Trace Elements in Human Nutrition*. WHO Technical Report Series No. 532. London: HMSO, 1973.

(ISBN 0 11 950617 3)

B A Fox and A G Cameron. *Food Science: a Chemical Approach*. 3rd ed. London: University of London Press, 1977.

(ISBN 0 34 021366 3)

S K Kon. *Milk and Milk Products in Human Nutrition*. FAO Nutritional Studies No. 27, 2nd revised ed. London: HMSO, 1972.

(ISBN 0 11 940438 9)

R A Lawrie. *Meat Science*. 2nd ed. Oxford: Pergamon, 1973.

(ISBN 0 08 017811 1)

Ministry of Agriculture, Fisheries and Food. *Food Standards Committee Report on Novel Protein Foods*. London: HMSO, 1974.

(ISBN 0 11 240829 X)

R B Duckworth. *Fruit and Vegetables*. Oxford: Pergamon, 1966.

(ISBN 0 08 011973 5)

N L Kent. *Technology of Cereals*. 2nd ed. Oxford: Pergamon, 1975.

(ISBN 0 08 018175 9)

Ministry of Agriculture, Fisheries and Food. *Food Standards Committee Second Report on Bread and Flour*. London: HMSO, 1974.

(ISBN 0 11 240828 1)

Department of Health and Social Security. *Recommended Daily Amounts of Food Energy and Nutrients for Groups of People in the United Kingdom*. (1979) Report on Health and Social Subjects No. 15. London HMSO, 1979.

(ISBN 0 11 320342 X)

US National Research Council. Food and Nutrition Board. *Recommended Dietary Allowances*. 8th revised ed. Washington: National Academy of Sciences, 1974.

(ISBN 0 30 902216 9)

Royal Society. *Metric Units, Conversion Factors and Nomenclature in Nutritional and Food Sciences.* Report of the Subcommittee on Metrication of the British National Committee for Nutritional Sciences. London: The Royal Society, 1972.

A A Paul and D A T Southgate. *McCance and Widdowson's The Composition of Foods,* 4th revised ed. Ministry of Agriculture, Fisheries and Food and Medical Research Council. London: HMSO, 1978.   (ISBN 0 11 450036 3)

B K Watt and A L Merrill. *Composition of Foods: Raw, Processed, Prepared.* Agriculture Handbook No. 8. Washington: US Department of Agriculture, 1963.

Index

Printed in England for Her Majesty's Stationery Office
by Hobbs the Printers of Southampton
(948) Dd717619 C100 6/82 G3313